The Weight Less Mind™

Why Diets Fail
The truth behind overeating

Acknowledgements

I feel blessed that I grew up with such amazing parents and such a beautiful sister. I love you all infinitely. Mum, Dad and Virginia, thank you for believing in me.

Mum, you have worked tirelessly to help this book come to fruition in time. Thanks so much for your patience and comprehension for my special work.

Thanks to all of my clients and workshops participants for your invaluable input.

About the Author

Georgia Foster has been working as a Clinical Hypnotherapist and Voice Dialogue Trainer for over 10 years in London, United Kingdom. Originally from Melbourne, Australia, her personal experience with low esteem and food issues led to years of self exploration to find answers. This book represents an outline of her personal journey and her successful work with thousands of people.

Georgia previously co-wrote *Slim By Suggestion*™ with Thorsons, 2001

Georgia Foster asserts the moral right to be identified as the author of this work

The Weight Less Mind™ is a trademark of Georgia Foster's

© Georgia Foster 2005

Typeset by Steve Verity (Fever Design)

Foster publishing 2005
Reprinted September 2005, Reprinted February 2008

Music composed by Nick Crofts

CD produced by Sound Recording Technology, 01480 461 880

ISBN 978-1-903607-61-9

A catalogue record for this book is available from the British Library

Printed in Great Britain by the MPG Books Group,
Bodmin and King's Lynn

Contents

Chapter 1

This is not a Diet Book

How I came to be where I am now

I would like you to know that one of my greatest gifts to you is this book. I feel very passionate about the work I do and how I came to be writing this now.

I was never an overweight child, but when I hit puberty I noticed that how you looked was extremely important. I was not your typical 'Aussie Blonde Beach Babe'. In fact, I was the opposite and the more I knew I was the opposite, the more I felt different and isolated. I started to use food as way to deal with life. People commented on the fact that I had puppy fat and that I would grow out of it, but I never did! All of my friends were slim and as my teenage years went on, so did the weight. I dieted on and off but each time I gained the weight, the lower my self esteem became.

The relationships I attracted didn't help either. I had way too many boyfriends who chiselled away at what self esteem I had left, but then I didn't feel I could get anybody better anyway. I really thought I was a second class citizen in life. I thought everybody was better, cleverer and more attractive than me.

When I was 24 I ran away for two weeks from my job, my family and my friends. Looking back, I realise now that I was heading for a breakdown. I ran away to a health farm that specialised in emotional wellbeing rather than physical wellbeing. I wanted to find out who I really was. I was looking for answers that I felt I couldn't find at home. After a week, I was surprised to see that there were other people who felt exactly like I did. I was relieved that, like me, they disliked themselves too. I didn't at that time have the answers but I was determined to find out what they were. I made a commitment to myself that I was going to search until I found some sort of peace in my own mind and body. I felt I was on a journey that I had no choice but to continue.

In 1994 I left Melbourne, Australia at the age of 28 to discover who I really was.

I went to California to train in a psychology theory called Voice Dialogue. This psychology theory changed my life. Voice Dialogue is a theory that Hal and Sidra Stone (both Jungian Psychologists) created. I had the great pleasure of studying with them and to this day I still talk about their work. The training I had with them has played a major part in the success of my clinic work and seminars.

After California, I went to London and studied for 18 months to be a clinical hypnotherapist. After I qualified, the college invited me back to lecture for them, which I did for 2 years. I saw through my own client base and the students that hypnosis was a wonderful tool to aid lack of confidence, stopping smoking and, of course, losing weight. I myself started losing weight, but not by dieting. I was miraculously losing weight simply by using my own techniques.

I was told by fellow lecturers that losing weight was the toughest of all of the therapies and yet I was getting great results, personally and professionally. My reputation for specialising in self esteem was helping people to lose weight and gain confidence, and this is where it all began.

This is not a diet book

Diets create stress through placing unrealistic demands and expectations upon us. We really want to succeed, and set out with good intentions to eat healthy food or restrict our food intake, only to find ourselves caught once again in what seems a never ending cycle of denial and binge.

Dieting is a nightmare - in fact, it is detrimental to our wellbeing. Detrimental because we do not understand why we keep repeating the denial and binge cycle: the consequence of this is that as we become disillusioned, we begin to dislike ourselves and sometimes the people around us.

To put it bluntly, we become angry and frustrated because we do not understand why we cannot keep to the bargain which we struck with ourselves to be healthier and therefore happier.

Eating out

Dining out is a dieter's nightmare, particularly when those we are dining with are not aware that we are on a diet. Or the people we are dining with are desensitised to our dieting because we have been trying 'this' or 'that' diet through the years they have known us. So they dismiss us with: "Oh, here she/he goes again." And the ironic fact is we dismiss ourselves. We continually set ourselves up for failure because diets are unrealistic and create stress.

Shopping

Buying new clothes is meant to be fun, even window shopping. But how many of us look at a window display and see those skinny, flat-stomached clothes dummies and compare ourselves to a plastic figure? We are not, thank heavens, plastic. We are living flesh and blood with hopes and dreams.

When we look at the display window, we catch our reflection in the glass and it is then, unfortunately, that we go into an overdrive of self-criticism, for we do not see our beauty: in our own mind we create a distorted view. The view we perceive is flawed and so we suck in our stomachs, curse our thighs and wish our lives away.

The Global Dieting Industry

The Hollywood regime of those oh-so-skinny stars with perfect makeup and gorgeous gowns can fuel our sense of inadequacy - so too does the advertising industry. Photos are air- brushed and naturally occurring rounder parts of the male and female anatomy are slimmed down. It is an industry made to sell perfection, and they are selling us the idea that we, too, can achieve the same outcome if we part with our money and buy their product.

This brings us to the big question: why are we not living our weight loss successfully? Why is the diet industry a multi billion pound business? Because the media and corporations have educated us that if we eat a little less and exercise a little more, then we lose weight. While this is correct to a certain degree, the question remains - if it is that simple why do we put all the weight we have lost back on again and into the bargain possibly gain extra weight, weight we did not have before?

Why is the dieting business so huge? (No pun intended.) It's because this type of reasoning about weight loss does not work for many people and this is why people are constantly searching for the miracle diet, and when one diet fails they search for another. Of course there are success stories, but the fact is that there is money to be made out of dieting and therefore it is big business.

If losing weight was about food and exercise alone, the dieting fad would have died out long ago because everybody would have achieved their desired weight loss the first time around and kept the weight off.

The truth is, even the most beautiful people in this world are continually dieting to achieve what they consider perfection.

Binge Eating

Every one of us has binge eaten at some point in our life and we have done so because we either needed to feel comforted or alternatively we've over-extended our stomach on sinful food because it tasted so good. By this I mean we may dine at an expensive restaurant which has a speciality dish, and though we are aware that we are stretching our stomachs beyond comfortable capacity, we order that speciality dish. We tell ourselves in both cases that: "It doesn't matter, not this once." We won't do it again. These are very different forms of binge eating. However, both originate from the desire to enjoy the sensation and comfort of food in the mouth.

Over the few next pages I will take you into a new territory where you will discover why your eating patterns continue to place you under stress, and from this you will gain an understanding of how and why these patterns have occurred. Then you will be further equipped for the future through the benefits of the enclosed CD.

June – Case Study

June phoned as she had read an article about the success of one of my clients in a monthly magazine. She said what attracted her to my work is that I do not believe in diets. For some of you who have been on the diet treadmill for many years like I was, you will recognise the attraction of this concept. June asked me if I provided pills if there was no diet. I replied, "No, you don't need pills. It's about changing your attitude towards yourself, gaining self esteem and developing coping mechanisms that have nothing to do with food." Down the phone I could hear June's brain ticking over: she liked this idea and promptly made an appointment.

A week later, June entered my consulting room. She was a very shy woman in her late forties, who had spent her life looking after two children and her husband while working full time as a social worker.

June had been on every diet known to mankind. Like all dieters she had, over 20 years, lost a lot of weight, gained a lot of weight and was at the end of her tether.

June described her life as one big diet. She said her husband rolled his eyes, bored of the whole dieting concept. He kept telling her: "Maybe you're just meant to be overweight." This just made June feel more and more determined and more and more insecure. She said she felt such a failure. Her tears of frustration and anger were followed by a very common question. "Why can't I lose weight successfully? I am so hopeless. I loathe my body. I feel so out of control with food. I'm either on a diet or overeating. I am a very busy person and yet I am constantly thinking about food. From the moment I wake up in the morning till when I go to bed at night I am thinking about food. I feel like I am going crazy. If my thoughts were radioed to the outside world, they would think I was barking mad."

Stress = Food

The more I learned about June's life, the more I realised that June ate purely to deal with stress. When I first explained to her that her problem wasn't food but it was stress, she looked at me as if I was a little odd for a few moments. So I explained to her that food was the symptom, not the cause, of her weight issues and if it really was as simple as going on a diet on a Monday with a goal of losing 32 pounds we all would have done it and got on with our lives.

June's habit of overeating had been a 20 year cycle as she moved between the biscuit tin at work through to cooking huge meals for her two sons and husband every evening, and during this process she had lost any concept of what real hunger felt like. June's trigger to eat had nothing to do with being hungry, her trigger was stress.

As a social worker, June continually listened to and dealt with other people's problems during the day, and then in the evening she returned home and continued working as mother and wife while dealing with any problems her family might have incurred during their day. Her only way to cope with this stressful way of life was with food.

June had literally trained her mind over many years that the only way to cope with everyday life was to overeat. So it is no wonder that when she dieted, she failed after a few weeks because she was not dealing with her stress.

When June was losing weight she was delighted, but she had never dealt with her emotional stress and so she would put the weight back on. Put plainly, her emotional stress when dieting had nowhere else to go. Her unconscious mind got confused because stress = food and ultimately that is what happened - she would start overeating again.

Unknowingly, June's emotional stress had led her down the path to low self worth and a sense of no self control.

Fortunately, with the help of our hypnosis sessions and through listening to the self hypnosis CD which I provided, June was able to train herself to recognise when her emotional stress kicked in, and she learned to value this valid emotion of stress rather than automatically stuffing it down with food.

June's whole world opened up when she realised her weight gain wasn't about food, but about recognising and dealing with the underlying issues of stress. The consequence of this is that June moved on, losing a lot of weight which she has kept off.

June's positive outcome is a typical result of the work I do.

So if it's not about dieting, then what is it about?

Throughout this book you will meet people like June who deal with life's issues through food, and more than likely you may identify with some. This book is about re-training your mind so you can learn to manage your emotions by other, more appropriate methods than food.

Each chapter in this book will give you tools to show and guide you out of the self-loathing and self-abusive relationship you have with yourself. This may sound harsh, but how we actually think and therefore feel about ourselves is the core to all of these emotions. The old statement: 'Treat yourself like you would your best friend' is indeed true, for when you think about it, how many of us actually do treat ourselves with the love and respect we give to a close friend?

The Radio Crazy Syndrome

You may not have consciously thought about how you actually talk to yourself until this book, but we are all talking to ourselves all of the time. Talking to ourselves is a normal activity; however, often it is to the detriment of your self esteem and self belief. To the outside world our inner chatter is silent, but internally how we talk to ourselves can be like radio crazy.

The following is a list of questions that are representative of the radio crazy thoughts that go through many of my clients' minds.

1. Do you wake up in the morning and the first thing you think about is food?
2. Are you surprised that no matter how busy you are, food is on your mind?
3. Do you feel isolated from other people because you are overweight?
4. Do certain situations or people trigger a binge?
5. Do you recognise real hunger?
6. Do you feel like you are going mad because you are either thinking about dieting or food all the time?
7. Do you feel anxious about eating in front of other people?
8. Do you overeat when you are alone?
9. Do you get angry with other people when they are successful at losing weight?
10. Do you eat to avoid certain confrontations?
11. Do you keep your weight on to avoid getting on with certain areas of your life?
12. Do you avoid sexual contact because you feel you are too self conscious about your weight?
13. Do you have an overweight uniform that you wear because you can't bear the thought of buying new clothes at your size?
14. Are you in fear of looking in shop windows and mirrors?
15. Do you dread going on holiday because of your weight?

If you answered yes to any or all of these questions, it is simply demonstrating how much your radio crazy has become a habit. Being overweight can often lead to emotional isolation, loneliness and depression. Overweight people are too scared to talk about it to anyone because they are worried that if they did, people would think they were going mad. Slim people just think: "Why don't they just get on with it?" so keeping quiet is the best solution, as well as secretly overeating.

Constantly thinking about food has become a normal way of life. It may sound strange, but your mind has trained itself to think this way. In fact, it thinks this is how you deal with life – by food, whether you are thinking about it or eating it.

One of my many radio crazy stories

I lived for a number of years with models. They all were tall, glamorous and could eat whatever they wanted without gaining weight. I, on the other hand, was constantly struggling with food and my weight. I tortured myself every day by either starving myself or bingeing. There seemed to be no in-between. One of their friends came over for a barbecue one day and suggested that if I lost weight, how much more attractive I would be. She then went on to say, why didn't I just exercise a little more and eat less? Not only did she say it in front of friends and family, but my new boyfriend. I was mortified. If there had been a hole I would have gladly gone down it with my bag of biscuits, cheese and a bottle of wine just to finish myself off. My boyfriend then kindly suggested that going on a diet would be a good thing because I would feel so much better about myself. I remember thinking, "If only it were that simple." I felt so helpless, unworthy, dumb and seriously alone. Being overweight is such a lonely experience. The isolation is frightening and emotionally extremely destructive to your self esteem. The rollercoaster of emotions that overweight people and those with food issues go through is so underestimated.

Please note: you are not going crazy! It's just how you have trained your mind to think, feel and behave. Radio crazy is a trained habit, a habit that this book will show you can be dealt with, so you can start to have a wonderful, supportive, relaxing radio station playing in your head.

Self Improvement

Over the course of reading this book and listening to the CD, you will start to notice that you are no longer berating yourself as much and that you have more peace in your mind and body. As your self esteem is improving, so will your attitude towards food. Physically, you will start to release the weight because emotionally you don't need it anymore.

To see this is wonderful, but to experience it is even better. Radio crazy can start to become a thing of the past. In a later chapter we will talk more about this, but for now just trust that the process of change is your right. Everybody has the right to like themselves, including you! The more you start to believe this, the more the weight will drop away. If you do not have weight to lose but binge or are bulimic, you will start to notice the self disgust is starting to lose momentum because you don't need to eat food for emotional reasons. That is why this book is not about dieting.

Food is your choice

If you wish to follow a particular eating programme, that is your choice. You must first consult your doctor. I am not a nutritionist and do not claim to be an adviser on what to eat, but one thing I do know is that eating the freshest food will enhance your metabolism, energy, health and wellbeing. So if you can incorporate 'real food' such as fish, chicken, red meat, vegetables, fruit and rice your body will thank you even more.

Your Positive Radio Station

The questions I asked previously are, as I said, made up of some of the most common radio crazy statements. So what if you could change these comments? You can. You see, these comments relate to a state of mind. You can train your mind and body to be healthy and happy with your weight. Being slim is a habit you can learn.

The following statements are the flipside of the previous questions that clients comment after a workshop or coming to see me privately.

1. I wake up in the morning and feel a sense of emotional freedom about food.
2. My day is full of many different things to do and food is just a part of it, not all of it.
3. I don't worry about what other people think of my weight. I am doing the best job possible with the right emotional tools now.
4. I realise that my mother was one of my triggers to overeating

and now I am assertive with her and myself. I am taking responsibility for my own relationship with food, rather than blaming situations and others.

5. I now enjoy the real feeling of hunger and enjoy the fact that I can safely leave food on my plate when I know I have had enough.

6. I do not have the same anxiety about losing weight. It is now a safe experience and my radio crazy supports me rather than works against me.

7. I feel liberated that I can eat in front of slim people without the anxiety.

8. When I am alone I now enjoy my own company rather than the company of food.

9. Other people have the right to lose weight successfully just as I do.

10. I now realise that overeating only exacerbates avoidance and in the end I am the only one who loses out.

11. Staying overweight is not supporting me any more. I have the right to be successful at whatever I do.

12. I feel much more relaxed about myself as a sexual being. I am now enjoying being intimate. It has improved the quality of my relationship.

13. I feel really excited that I am wearing clothes that make me feel good about myself.

14. When I look at myself I see the slim, confident person that I deserve to be.

15. I am so looking forward to this holiday because I feel so much better in myself physically and emotionally.

In the chapter 'Why Hypnosis Works' you will discover that the above statements can be yours. I am sure there are many other statements you would like to feel are a part of your everyday life. Statements that support your true desire to be successful at losing weight. We will explore those statements and many more as we go along.

The enclosed CD

By the end of chapter 3, you will be ready to listen to track 1. Chapter 3 explains in great detail the power of your mind and its incredible ability to change your relationship with yourself and with food.

Chapter 2

Inner Dialogue

The Inner Dialogue method is part of my personal and professional daily life. I live by the tools and techniques in this book, as do my clients.

Inner Dialogue represents how we talk to ourselves internally. To the outside world we can hide this dialogue and we are thankful that people cannot read our minds. However, how we talk to ourselves is often of great disservice to our emotional wellbeing.

We are all made up of many parts or sub-personalities. These parts originally develop unconsciously when we are young to help us deal with life, then they became a habit. You may, for example, look at the dynamics of your family make-up and recognise that perhaps you were the child who kept the peace in the home, or perhaps you were the gregarious child who got away with a lot. Somewhere along the way, your mind decided that the best way of being loved was to develop certain personality traits. The aim of these personalities was protection against vulnerability. It works very well for many years, until you grow up and go into the big world outside and realise that sometimes these personality traits are a hindrance rather than helpful.

Case Study - Jane

Jane's weight had been an issue since leaving university. She had been on many diets over many years, and by the time she came to see me in Notting Hill she was extremely desperate. At the time Jane was thirty-two, single and working as an accountant in a large firm. She heard about my work through her neighbour who had been to one of my workshops.

Jane wanted a one to one appointment with me rather than a group, as she felt too self-conscious to discuss her weight issues with other people.

Jane grew up in a rough area of London. To protect herself, she was educated from a very young age not to look anybody in the eye and to keep her head down. Her parents argued frequently and young Jane soon learned in her home environment that staying quiet and not seeking attention was the safest experience. At school she was shy and had very few friends. The way Jane learned to cope with life was through reading, writing and school work. All these activities were quiet, low maintenance emotional tools. Jane had succeeded in her childhood in achieving what her parents wanted, attending university then qualifying as an accountant. On paper she was the crème de la crème of the university, and some of the best-known firms offered her a position as a trainee.

The outside world

It was a different story when Jane left the safe world of study and entered the outside corporate world. It was then, Jane said, she began to put on a lot of weight. We discussed what she thought had changed emotionally for her. She pondered over this for a while as I discussed the inner dialogue theory with her and then something in Jane clicked. Jane told me she was not a popular person at work. Her boss had accused her of being aloof. It was difficult for her to make friends because she could not make eye contact. People thought she was weird and stayed away from her.

As a child, being aloof had kept her safe but as an adult, Jane's aloofness was stirring up pure rejection. Her mind was confused. Her aloofness personality trait that had worked in the past was creating problems. We discussed what we could do.

Scanning the past

Jane's mind scanned her past and she saw for herself that food was the answer. It had become an unconscious habit. She was stuffing down her feelings of rejection with food, and at the same time her weight was going up and her self esteem was going down.

Jane's inner dialogue was saying, "Nobody likes you. You're a hopeless case. You can't even manage a day without bingeing on chocolate. You've ruined this week now by what you have eaten, you may as well just continue bingeing until Monday." and at the same time, Jane's inner dialogue was also telling her, "Don't get close, you'll get hurt. Stay a distance away. People are only trouble." The aloof part had become her strongest personality trait along with the overweight, inner critical part. They had become her inner protective team.

The sad thing was that Jane desperately wanted to belong. She wanted to know what it was like to have real friends and yet her unconscious personality trait kept her from achieving this.

Developing the confident part

In order for Jane to lose weight, it was clear that she needed to develop a personality trait that was confident, warm and open. This part or sub-personality had always been there; however, it had become suppressed as a result of Jane's upbringing. This suppressed part of Jane's mind had told her as a child: "Don't go there, you will only get hurt. It's unsafe."

Jane liked the idea that she could start to become confident and yet at the same time, through her lifetime of aloofness, it seemed very foreign to her. By now she understood that food was the symptom, not the cause, of her weight, and that by educating her mind through the CD she could develop this part to be present in her daily life, and slowly but surely she began to develop her confident, warm, open part. This was accomplished through what I call baby steps.

It takes practice, but the bottom line was and is: Jane deserves to be happy with herself. Why should she continue to live a life of suffering through this state of mind? Why should she always feel an outsider when she didn't have to be? It was an emotional habit, a habit that Jane now knows is out of date.

Jane is now enjoying her life mixing and socialising more confidently as a slim person.

Decisions

The Inner Dialogue is about breaking down the inner conversations you have with yourself. It is important to find out what parts you have created that support your adult life and the ones that don't. By exploring this, you can start to make better decisions about what is right for you now rather than what was right for you all those years ago. It is about recognising what is really true for you and what is not.

At the present time this may seem daunting, but over the next few chapters you will learn about these inner voices/parts that you have trained to work against you and your best made plans.

The Slim Confident Part

When we make a decision to do something, the motivation comes from one or more inner voices. Even if we don't get around to following through and doing it, the thought was there which triggered a spark from within, like a fire of energy. When we do follow through, it is this energy which spurs us on to achieve something that is important to us.

An example of one of these sparks is the voice of the Slim Confident part. You would have experienced this spark as a moment of inspiration and motivation when you heard about this book or when you found it in a bookshop.

This part is the inner voice that 100 per cent really wants you to lose weight. Your Slim Confident part has the resources to show you and to guide you on how to look after yourself. The important question now is: "If I have this Slim Confident part, why doesn't it hang around to help me continue to lose weight?"

Example 1

Katie attended one of my 2 day workshops a few months ago. On her assessment form she wrote that yo-yo dieting was part of her life. She had formed a habit of going on a diet and being very successful for 3 weeks, and then she would go on a massive binge and put the weight on again. Katie repeated this cycle again and again.

Example 2

Jennifer had a similar problem. She would go on a diet with the goal of losing 1½ stones, then she would binge eat and put the weight back on. Jennifer's goal was to go from 11 stones to 9 stones, but that last ½ stone was always a mystery. She would lose 1 stone but get stuck at that weight which she would maintain for a while but then put the stone she had lost back on again.

We will talk more about Katie and Jennifer later, but for now it is clear that they do know how to lose weight. It is irrelevant whether it is 3 weeks or 1½ stones. Katie's and Jennifer's minds do know how to bring in the Slim Confident part. The question is: why does the Slim Confident part disappear when they are at a crucial point of their weight loss regime?

If everybody knows what to eat, how much to eat, how to exercise and ultimately lose weight, why can't they maintain this process and get on with their lives? What is the resistance?

The Inner Critic

I am going to introduce the part that I spend most of my clinic time with, and it is the part that I used to spend most of my inner dialogue time with.

I want to share with you some of my own (fortunately now out of date) inner dialogue that I shifted physically and emotionally by the techniques in this book.

- What's the point in losing weight? I'm just going to put it on again and some more.
- My stomach is huge, I look pregnant.
- My boyfriend is with me because he cannot find anybody else to love him.
- I am with my boyfriend because no-one else will love me.
- I want to become bulimic. At least then I could maintain my weight. It's a way to control my out of control eating.
- Everybody is commenting about my weight behind my back.
- I'll never amount to anything. Let's face it, if I can't even lose weight how will I ever manage everything else?
- It's hopeless.
- I'm so bored of thinking about my weight. Why can't I think about anything else?
- None of my family are overweight. What is my problem?

- I detest myself. Is this how I am going to be for the rest of my life? The thought of going on like this makes me so sad and depressed.

Sound familiar?

I could go on for a whole book on how much I used to beat myself up. To the outside world I was a calm, happy and popular person, but on the inside I was miserable, dissatisfied and filled with self loathing. I was disgusted with myself. I actually hated myself. I couldn't believe that I had to wake up with myself every god damn day. You may think this is harsh, but this type of inner dialogue is common amongst people who have a history of struggling with their weight and their relationship with food.

On becoming a therapist in 1994, I realised that how I talked to myself was exactly the same as the next client who walked in the door. They didn't all have weight issues, but predominately what holds a person back is their own inner dialogue with themselves. You see, the previous statements I believed were true of myself. I thought that my own inner conversations with myself were a true reflection of who I was as a whole person. I believed that this was what everybody else thought of me. I was filled with self loathing because this is what I thought about myself and therefore what hope I did I have?

Elephant with pink spots

When I studied hypnotherapy, I realised that how I spoke to myself was a habit, a habit that I had the power to change. A habit that, at the time, seemed daunting and almost too much to bear; however, I recognised that because I believed these inner conversations to be true, they were true! The way I thought about myself became a self fulfilling prophecy. It's like asking someone not to think about an elephant with pink spots. My whole life revolved around giving myself a hard time. With the help of hypnotherapy, I started to work more deeply on these thoughts and the inner conversations I had with myself and I began to notice real changes, first of all in how I talked to myself and secondly that food wasn't the epicentre of my life.

The Inner Critic part is a personality trait. It is the part that judges you and criticises you. It is the part that actually was created to protect you, and yet through a lifetime of experiences it has trained itself to work against you.

My Inner Critic statements are representative of the typical dialogue that overweight people have with themselves. Over my many years of being a therapist, it would be safe to say that I have heard pretty much every Inner Critic comment from people from all walks of life.

Silent but violent

If you purchased this book because you want to lose weight or change your relationship with food, you may recognise some of this behaviour. You may have other dialogue going on in your mind that has nothing to do with weight or food. Let's face it: all of us are talking to ourselves all of the time and this talk is often silent and violent.

The point is, how we talk to ourselves is a learned behaviour. How we talk to ourselves is a habit, a habit that we can change.

The mind works by recalling from your memory bank any experience that you have already stored that looks like, or is similar to, something you are about to do.

Katie's Story

Katie, who I mentioned before, struggled to get past 3 weeks of dieting. Her unconscious mind had trained itself to think 3 weeks of dieting equalled stop. Somewhere in Katie's past, she had stopped dieting at 3 weeks. The cause of this could have been a change of job or perhaps a broken relationship, where her mind stopped her from dieting because it was emotionally unsafe at that particular time. Actually it is irrelevant what happened, but the fact is, her mind at 3 weeks had trained itself to stop at that point. This result was Katie felt down, and low self worth started to build within her.

But it wasn't Katie who stopped losing weight after 3 weeks - it was her Inner Critic. Her Inner Critic scanned her mind and said, "Oops, 3 weeks - the last time you lost weight it got difficult at this stage." It started telling her, "Katie, it's getting too hard now. What about the party you're going to on Saturday night? You know you will blow it. You know you can't get past 3 weeks." And on and on the Inner Critic goes, as I said, like radio crazy.

At this point, Katie's Inner Critic begins to challenge her even more by suggesting that perhaps she should go down to the local shop and by a chocolate bar, just to tide her over. The Inner Critic thinks that this is the way to stop her from continuing to lose weight, because the Inner Critic thinks it is unsafe to go past 3 weeks. The more Katie tries to ignore these Inner Critic comments, the stronger they become - its voice starts to get stronger and stronger so that Katie finally has to give in and go to the shop to buy the chocolate bar. The worst thing is, the Inner Critic will then say to her, "I knew you couldn't do it - it didn't take long for you to fall off the dieting wagon." And so Katie's self loathing becomes stronger and even more powerful, so that she will then start to binge eat anything and everything that she can find.

The result of this is that Katie doesn't go to the party. She feels too guilty, too fat and too out of control. Her Inner Critic thinks on behalf of her and tells her everybody secretly knows that she binges and that she can't control her eating. This recent binge then just adds to her unconscious mind's library that dieting is unsafe, until the next time she finds a new diet in a magazine and then the treadmill starts all over again.

Katie's Inner Critic has become her strongest personality trait, to the detriment of her self worth.

This case study might seem cruel, but it is a typical case study of the issues my clients deal with every day.

The Inner Critic Rules

1. It knows everything about you, from your odd sexual thoughts to the cellulite on your thighs, and it will remind you just as you are about to make love to the person of your dreams.

2. It remembers even the most old, out of date information such as when you stole a pen from a department store when you were 10, and it will remind you of this out of date information just when you are just about to go for that all-important interview as the Sales Director of a department store.

3. It knows every time you have felt vulnerable, such as an unsuccessful diet, and will keep reminding you of this over and over so you don't try and do it again.

4. It reads other people's minds for you. It's like your own personal psychic.

5. It will hound you day in and day out until you give into its demands because it is frightened that if you don't listen to it, it will have failed its job and, of course, you listen.

6. It thinks that everybody else deals with their life much better than you do and it will constantly compare you to anybody and everybody in any situation where you feel slightly vulnerable, making you feel extremely vulnerable.

7. It is the part that loves procrastination and indecisiveness and prevents you from succeeding, because it has already played out the negative scene telling you that you will fail.

The truth is, the Inner Critic loves vulnerability. On any stirring or feeling that you have of being unsafe it is there in full force as a protective mechanism. It thinks if it gets in first then it is preparing you for the worst case scenario. If you listen to the Inner Critic it is guaranteed that you will be hesitant with your decision making. This lack of ability to make decisions leads to self doubt, often leaving the individual emotionally frozen, unable to pursue whatever it is that they truly want to do.

How to deal with the Inner Critic

The Inner Critic is there solely to criticise you and it always will. The question is how to deal with it.

The Slim Confident part represents the opposite part to the Inner Critic. It is the part that starts off well with all the best intentions, but once the Inner Critic kicks in with its own powerful comments it suppresses the Slim Confident part. Then this in itself becomes an unconscious habit; meanwhile the conscious mind doesn't understand - in other words, it doesn't get it. The conscious mind thinks you are going crazy.

After you have read chapter 3 you will be ready to listen to track 1 of the CD. Your mind will start to create for itself the library of how to lose weight by working with your inner dialogue rather than just the Inner Critic. You will never be able to lose your Inner Critic - if you try, it will just come back more violently than before. I have seen many participants in my workshops and my clinic work whose Inner Critic has been so powerful that it has led to depression. A lot of depression is based on repeated Inner Critic comments going round and round and round. Comments like: "It's all too hard. What's the point?" Over a period of time the Inner Critic leads to low self worth and depression sets in. The Inner Critic is just one voice. You cannot run away from it. You must work with it so that it understands it is safe for you to lose weight and gain self esteem. Remember, it thinks that it knows best all the time but it doesn't.

Over the next few chapters, you will met some other parts that will help you understand the personality traits that you have created earlier in life in order to feel safe. These personality traits have real voices. As you begin to understand these different parts, you can start to break your old patterns of thought and create new ones.

It's nobody else's business that you want to lose weight

A little tip when it comes to losing weight. As mentioned before, the Inner Critic loves to see you fail and it loves to think it can read other people's minds. So a kind word from your Slim Confident part: don't tell other people you are doing this because if you do tell someone else, the Inner Critic comes in and sets you up for failure. They may roll their eyes and even if they don't, the Inner Critic will interpret it this way and feed in to your mind comments on their behalf - this will lead to a major Inner Critic attack and a binge session. Remember: your diet is nobody's business but your own!

If you do feel 100 per cent safe then by all means tell a partner, family member or friend. However, before you do confide in them ask yourself this important question: is telling them going to emotionally help you or hold you back?

While you are training your own mind to lose weight, the Inner Critic is also learning that it is safe for you to lose weight and that it can relax and let go. It does take practice but stick with it, because it is well worth it. You are worth it!

Chapter 3

Why Hypnosis Works

Hypnosis in your daily life

You may not be consciously aware until this chapter, but hypnosis is a natural state that we all enter many times each day. A lot of people I meet say, "I couldn't possibly be hypnotised." However, everybody is able to be hypnotised by themselves or, if you choose, by someone else. The hypnosis state is experienced when we daydream. For example, when we are on a train and we lose memory of the last five stops. It is a state where our conscious mind starts to move into the background, as the unconscious mind starts to come forward. As you drift into sleep you must pass through the hypnotic daydream state. You cannot go to sleep without this process.

As we fall asleep our breathing starts to slow down, our heart rate drops, our circulation slows down as well as our metabolic rate. This process can take approximately 5 to 20 minutes. During this stage we are in hypnosis. During this time we are highly receptive to new learning. It is a very creative time. A lot of new ideas, businesses and inventions have been created during this time.

The Unconscious Mind

The unconscious mind, which is also called the right brain, is an amazingly powerful tool. We use it every second of the day and night, without most of the time being aware of it. There are some important facts in this chapter that will help you to understand why you have created certain habits and behaviours, and that you have the tools to change the ones you want to change and enhance the ones you like, such as the Slim Confident part.

At the beginning of all of my workshops, I like to explain how the unconscious mind works to alleviate any misconceptions, but first I would like to demonstrate to you the role of this part of your mind.

Time

The unconscious mind has no concept of time. That is why, when we sleep at night, we are not aware of how long we have slept until we check our watches or bedside clock. If we were aware of the time that we had slept, we would be exhausted. The reason why we sleep is to rest the body and the conscious mind. The unconscious mind never stops working. It is available 24 hours a day and it is fully functioning even while you are sleeping.

Your Body

It manages all the bodily functions such as your heart beating, lungs breathing, digesting, processing and eliminating food without you thinking about it. How much your unconscious mind manages is almost incomprehensible. We just trust that this part of the mind knows what to do and we just let it get on with it.

Your Memory Bank

Every single moment of your life is stored in this part of your mind. The unconscious mind does not operate chronologically If you wanted to recall anything from 10 years ago, your mind would not go back through every day till it arrived at that particular moment. If this was the case, you would be spending a very long time sorting through your memory bank! It is able to pinpoint that time accurately and efficiently. An example of this would be if I mentioned my experience of seeing the Eiffel Tower in Paris. If you have had the pleasure of seeing this magnificent structure, your mind would be able to recall instantly your memories of the Eiffel Tower too. It could have been 20 years ago or yesterday. The point is, your mind locates any experience that you have stored pretty much instantly.

Everything is Real

The unconscious mind comprehends every experience as a real experience. Unlike the conscious mind where there is rationale and logic, this deeper part of your mind doesn't know the difference between imagination and reality. This is the most important point to remember when it comes to making positive changes. It is the core part of the success of hypnosis.

When you daydream, your conscious vision fades and your unconscious mind's vision of whatever you are imagining becomes real. You can see, feel and hear what that thought is about, even though, in reality, it is not really in front of you at all. When you stop daydreaming, your conscious mind acknowledges that you were daydreaming but your unconscious mind saw that experience as real.

All of our Senses are Positive and Negative

The unconscious mind works solely on emotions and memories. It uses one or more or all of the senses to recall any memories, whether good or bad. We immediately associate situations and places not just by our visual recall but by all of the senses. A great example would be the smell of baking bread. It sends me into a state of warmth, love and a feeling of being safe. I can go there now, immediately, as I am typing, and perhaps you too can recall what it's like to smell the bread baking. Perhaps you can hear the sound of the oven door opening and the bread tray being moved to the bench as the steam rises, the smell becoming stronger and more enjoyable as your taste buds start to salivate. Then the butter comes out and is slathered all over the bread and it starts to melt into every part of the fluffy, fresh, warm bread.

The opposite side of the above example could be that baking bread is associated with a controlling mother who worried about you eating too much and restricted you to only one piece. Therefore baking bread is associated with rules, restrictions and not feeling cared for. Walking past a bakery could be an emotionally disturbing experience for you, so much that you refuse to buy freshly baked bread at the local bakery or, in fact, eat bread at all. If this is so, then your mind has recalled instantly the most prominent example of how to deal with bread.

One Trial Learning

In therapy, some emotional habits can be described as one trial learning. This expression is used when a client has trained their unconscious mind by one powerfully emotionally charged experience. This experience leads to a behaviour that becomes an instant habit.

Sally's One Trial Learning

When Sally was 15, she saw her father leave her mother. Sally watched the pain her mother went through, and how her mother reacted was by food. When Sally was in her early 20s, her first real serious boyfriend broke up with her without any explanation. She was devastated. Her mind scanned her memory bank to find out how to deal with this rejection. Without any conscious interaction, her mind remembered that how her mother dealt with it was by food, so Sally then started to binge. It was immediate, unconscious and, at the time, very effective in reducing her emotional pain. This one experience then went on to become a habit.

The Unconscious Mind and Vulnerability

Sally is a classic example of how the unconscious mind works so efficiently when it comes to finding immediate emotional support.

The memory bank, or what I call the library, recalled what seemed right at the time using all of the senses. When the emotional experience is high, the mind will find the most powerful example of how to deal with the situation even if it is to the detriment of you. It is impersonal. It doesn't know the difference between positive and negative, it just knows what you have experienced.

The mind experiences the fight or flight, 'should I stay or should I run' scenario as the vulnerability is too high to stay put. The unconscious mind has to make a decision as to how to alleviate the vulnerability.

It could have been the opposite. Sally's mother could have stopped eating due to the anxiety, or even have turned to alcohol. Her mother could have dealt with it in a completely healthy way. However it was dealt with at the time, it was deemed right by the unconscious memories Sally had.

The 4 different Brain Waves

There are 4 different brain wave activities that we use throughout the day and night.

Beta

The Beta state is called the waking state, where the conscious mind is going about its daily life involving rational thinking. It is a logical state. An example would be buying a train ticket immediately because the timetable says there is a train in 3 minutes. The brain is working much more rapidly to achieve what you need to achieve in your daily life. The conscious mind is the most prominent part of the mind during this time.

We are conscious most of the day, but it is important to know that at some stage the unconscious mind has to absorb your daily experiences.

Alpha

The Alpha state is a half awake/half asleep state. It is when you daydream, or when you can't remember reading for the past 10 minutes. It's a time when your conscious mind is sending the information to the unconscious mind to be absorbed, stored, ready to be recalled at any time.

During this time the unconscious mind is very intuitive. It can be a time when you find answers to questions, resolve problems and find solutions.

We all need to daydream just as children do. Children between the ages of 7 and 14 are predominately in the alpha state. This is the last stage of learning to become more adult, make logical choices and develop a sense of self.

This is the lighter state, more awake than asleep, as you drift into sleep or the last stage of coming out of the sleep state.

Theta

Theta is an experience of a much deeper state. Some would describe it as a meditative state, where you are highly open to new ideas. It is an experience where you may feel you have fallen asleep. It is the last stage just before you drift into sleep or the first stage before Alpha.

From infancy to around 7 years of age, a child will be predominately experiencing this state. When you think about how much an infant has to learn to do, such as walking, talking and making sense of the world, imagine as an adult being able to enter this state on a regular basis. You can, and you are, by listening to the CD.

Delta

Delta is when you are completely asleep. This is when the day's experiences are updating themselves fully so you can wake feeling refreshed the next day. This is also the state you are in when you are under a general anaesthetic.

The Library

After having absorbed the scientific side of how the mind works, let's start to bring it together with the Inner Dialogue theory.

As we naturally go into hypnosis many times every day, by listening to the CD you can utilise this time by supportive messages that your mind will view as real and true. Your memory bank will start to store, in your library, these suggestions of who you are now rather than using the old, out of date information.

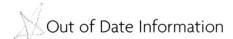 Out of Date Information

In the past, your mind was playing your own inner CD of radio crazy thinking: "Well, that's what we thought before and this is how we do things." Every time your mind thought, or should I say your Inner Critic said to you, "It's all too hard, I really want to go to this party this evening, I know I am going to blow it." your mind agrees with you because it takes this on board as a real, true statement. Just add a couple of similar statements already stored in your library, then your mind will think this is how to feel and behave. "Let's go to the party and blow it!" Your unconscious mind thinks this is normal, but your conscious mind does not understand. It gets totally frustrated with you as you do, too, and then the vicious cycle goes on and on. The radio crazy begins over and over again.

Your library is out of date, but can only be out of date when you replace it with information that reflects what you want to feel now and in the future. As the mind doesn't know the difference between reality and imagination, your mind, every time you listen to the CD, is affirming that your Inner Critic is comfortable with you losing weight. Your mind will be storing the fact that it is emotionally safe for you to have the Slim Confident part as your strongest voice rather than being suppressed by the Inner Critic.

In the previous example of Sally and rejection, by listening to the CD she was developing a choice of how to react that was supporting her conscious wishes. Sally's mind trained itself that rejection, unfortunately, is an experience that we all have from time to time, but that it doesn't mean rejection = food. The new library for Sally made perfect sense. Sally moved on and her relationship with food became healthy and emotionally safe.

Willpower

There is no such thing as lack of willpower. If you have consciously tried to lose weight or change your relationship with food to be healthier without success, it simply means your unconscious mind thinks this is normal. Your unconscious mind thinks that overeating is simply how you deal with life. When both parts of your mind are disagreeing, the unconscious mind will win the argument, because it thinks it is protecting you.

By reading this book and listening to the CD you can educate both parts of your mind to work together, rather being opposing forces.

Repetition

If there is one thing I stipulate over and over and over again to my clients, this is it. Your inner library, at present, represents every failure at losing weight. The only way to combat this is to build your new library with the opposite information. The more you listen to your CD, the stronger it will become. The repetition is extremely important, and those who listen to the CD every day or, at worst, every other day will experience much more effective results.

The more you listen to the CD the stronger the library becomes, so much so that you will not question your self esteem improving, it will just become a habit. As your self esteem is improving, your relationship with food will too. You won't want to overeat because the library thinks that is 'old hat' because it is. It is an old way of thinking that you have moved on from. Emotionally, you will find that the CD is helping you sleep, to de-stress and to have time simply to look after you. I call it Me Time. It is 20 minutes in your day when you are doing something positive for you.

The Enclosed CD

The enclosed CD has 3 tracks. You can start to listen to track 1 now. You need to make sure that you are sitting or lying down, feeling warm and safe. You must be stationary throughout the CD. If you need to wake at any time you can, by simply opening your eyes.

Before you start to listen to the CD, I would like to explain how it works. A lot of people have many misconceptions about what it is meant to feel like. Following are the most common questions. I hope I answer all of them for you.

Some common questions about the CD:

1. *Will I fall asleep? Some people do fall asleep. This will not change the results of the self hypnosis. Remember, the information is still going in. The unconscious mind is open 24 hours a day.*

2. *When is the best time to listen to it? The best time is before you go to sleep, but often if my client does not want their partner to know (which is very common, and the next chapter will explain why), then perhaps at lunchtime in a board room, or when you know you will not be disturbed. Some people love waking up to the CD and feel that it sets them up for the day. A little tip: if your binge time is when you get home from work while preparing food, you can pop the CD on as soon as you get in. This will start to break the habit of eating between meals. In fact, you can pop the CD on whenever you are feeling down, negative or having a panic attack about your relationship with food. It will really help to put things into a healthier perspective.*

3. *If I am interrupted during it, does it mean it hasn't worked? No, not at all. It just means that you haven't completed the CD track, so maybe try it again later.*

4. *Can other people listen to the CD? No, tell them to go and buy their own book! You made the effort, you spent the money, so can they if they are serious about it!*

5. *What if I fall asleep and listen to all of the tracks? Fantastic! Not essential, but a big blast of hypnosis is brilliant for anybody. It will only enhance your progress.*

6. *If my mind is busy is it still working? Yes, absolutely. It doesn't make any difference. You will, on some level, be absorbing the information. It will also help you to relax.*

7. *If I move around will it bring me out of hypnosis? No, just move around if you need to during the CD. A lot of people, when they are relaxed, recognise how much tension they hold in their body, so any adjustments are beneficial. If you want to cough, scratch or sneeze it will not make any difference.*

Now you can start to listen to track 1.

Points to remember:

- You have the right to lose weight and maintain a healthy weight.
- You are now starting to build a new library of information that is supporting you rather than working against you.
- Your mind understands now that by listening to track 1 of the CD you are on your way to the real, slim you.

Chapter 4

The Pleaser

What is The Pleaser?

Whenever I introduce the Pleaser to workshop participants I notice awkward smiles appear on many faces and I can identify with these awkward smiles, for the Pleaser part is a part that is close to my own heart. It was, and still is, one of my strongest parts. On the positive side, I have to say 'Thanks' to my Pleaser for being my front-of-house personality, because it led me to this profession. However, the negative side of my Pleaser led me to many years of self-loathing and binge eating.

You can spot a Pleaser a mile away because they are always willing to do things that often other people are not.

Questionnaire:

1. Do you over-commit to keep everybody happy?
2. Do you feel guilty if you say 'No' to people?
3. Do you play over in your mind what you previously said, worrying that you might have offended someone?

4. Do you keep the conversation going to avoid silences?
5. Do you worry about not being liked?
6. Do you have a lot of acquaintances?
7. Do friends dump their problems onto you, knowing that you will pick up the pieces?
8. If somebody does something awful to you, do you say it's OK when really you want to give them a piece of your mind?

The Pleaser and Fear

The Pleaser is the part that harbours the emotions of guilt, fear and abandonment.

When I discovered that I had a strong Pleaser, I realised how much of a doormat I had become through most of my life. So shocked was I by this discovery that at one stage I considered naming my self esteem book 'I used to be a Doormat' because I realised that the Pleaser controlled my emotions and therefore restricted my relationships with family and friends.

The purpose of the Pleaser is to keep everybody else happy. It is the part that makes sure everybody else's needs are met first. Of all of the parts, it is this part that has the strongest link to emotional eating.

The Pleaser personality is often charming, open and warm to the outside world. It is a very attractive character trait to have, because you will be well liked. The down side is: the more you look after someone else, the less time you have to look after you.

I don't know whether you have heard the saying 'fat people are jolly'? Well, fat people pretend to be jolly. I don't know every overweight person in this world, but the ones I have met kept their Pleaser façade up so they keep everybody else happy through entertaining them. I am not suggesting slim people are not entertaining, but people with a strong Pleaser who have weight issues will more than likely be the life and soul of the party, because they want to make sure everybody is enjoying themselves. Pleasers go out of their way to make sure everyone has a drink and that anybody who looks like they are being left out will be nurtured with attention. The result is that everybody loves the party Pleaser.

Pleasers are lovely people because they are good listeners and will always entertain the idea of co-ordinating other people's lives because they need to be useful. The shame of it is that by keeping busy pleasing others, the Pleaser has no time left energetically or emotionally for pleasing themselves.

The word 'NO'

Most people love having a Pleaser person in their lives because they do the things that the person doesn't like doing. Pleasers say 'Yes' to everything because they are frightened that if they say 'No' they will be rejected. The irony of this is that, deep down, the fear of being rejected is actually more important to the Pleaser than the person they are pleasing, and this is the reason they say 'Yes'.

If they say 'No', their Pleaser will say, internally, "That person is offended" or "If you don't say yes, they may not ask you again and then you won't have any friends".

The word 'No' stirs too many fearful emotions in the Pleaser: the emotions of rejection, abandonment and being left out.

Pleaser Case Study

In the Weight Less Mind™ workshop I spend time with my clients discussing Inner Dialogue and its implications relating to weight issues. One of these workshops was attended by Jane, aged 54, who was a classic Pleaser. During the discussion about the Inner Dialogue theory, Jane couldn't stop laughing and I sensed that she was uncomfortable with the subject because it was stirring up within her a realisation that the Pleaser was controlling her life. Jane called me a few days later and this is what she said:

"I was shocked to learn my whole life I have run around looking after other people. On one hand I feel relieved that at least now I have a method of moving out of this Pleaser state, but I feel also very sad that I've spent my whole life running around looking after everybody else to the detriment of my personal and professional life. I feel I have wasted my life."

Jane's image to the outside world was of a person who was always there for others. She was godmother to many of her friends' children, so she was constantly rushing here and rushing there trying to keep everybody happy.

In addition to this, Jane had looked after her ill mother most of her adult life. Every holiday, she took her mother with her and during the week she spent two evenings as well as every Sunday with her, the result being that her mother expected this. Jane felt guilty if she had to work late and missed an evening visit, so she gave up her successful but demanding job for a less stressful one. The end result of all this Pleaser juggling was that Jane was emotionally and physically bankrupt. No wonder she felt she had wasted her life.

The feeling of having missed out on life is quite common to many Pleaser people and the discovery of this can be a highly emotional experience. Perhaps you can identify with this and, if you do, it means that you now have the opportunity to move out of this state and start to value yourself.

Care and nurturing of Self

I suggested to Jane that she start practising taking care of and nurturing herself. By this I told her that she had to learn to put her own needs first, in other words to be more selfish with how she allocated her time. "Other people do it and get away with it, why not you?" I stated. At first, this seemed a monumental task to Jane because when a Pleaser starts to please themselves it changes the relationship dynamics of the people around them.

Little by little, Jane learned how to set boundaries on her Pleaser, beginning with her mother. She explained to her mother how exhausted she was and that she would spend one evening a week with her instead of two.

As it turned out this was an equitable arrangement for both, as Jane's mother respected her decision and this increased Jane's confidence to set boundaries by saying 'No' when the situation was not agreeable to her. Interestingly, Jane decided to spend her free evening doing what she had always wanted to do: she enrolled in an art class.

The Pleaser and the people around you

When a person begins to work with their Pleaser it can have an interesting effect which could be likened to throwing a pebble into a lake, and through this action circles radiate out.

The group at a two day workshop in Edinburgh a few months ago included a mother called Ruth and her daughter called Penny. I have no objection to family or close friends attending my workshops together; however, often one or both parties may feel inhibited in talking or expressing themselves. They may feel they cannot relax as much as they want to for fear of being judged (another common Pleaser trait). The two women were lovely. Ruth was 66 at the time and on the first day she did not say a word, just stared at me for the whole day. During the hypnosis, she sat tight as a ball in her chair whereas the rest of the group chilled out and relaxed on the carpet. I never had an issue with Ruth doing this because I could see she was feeling uncomfortable.

The following Saturday, I was back in Edinburgh for the second day of the workshop and I could not believe my eyes. There in the group was a glowing Ruth raving about the CD and how food was no longer an issue. Through listening to the CD, she had become aware of why she was eating and now ate only when she was hungry. She then explained how she had begun to stand up to her controlling husband for she realised within herself that she wanted to get on with her own life. Ruth said she hadn't realised how much she had put her husband's needs first and her own needs last: now she felt that she wanted to make more of her life as well as her relationships with other people. I admired Ruth's newly acquired strength to make these changes, and hoped her husband would make some compromises so Ruth would continue to blossom and their relationship would grow.

Three months later, Ruth's daughter Penny, who was also on the course, emailed me to say that she had lost 21 pounds since the workshop and how delighted she was that food was no longer an issue - she would treat herself when she felt like it but, on the whole, life was just so much easier. Penny then continued, "I feel like the weight has come off my mind. It seems odd that I don't have this stress when the children leave their food. I don't have to eat it anymore. I just put it straight into the bin." I replied to Penny thanking her for her email, and asked how her mother was getting along. I had often thought about Ruth and Penny and had visions of Ruth doing a Shirley Valentine! Penny replied that a few weeks after the course, Ruth's husband had banned her from listening to the CD. My heart sank. Penny wrote that Ruth had retreated back into her old ways to appease her husband. He told her 'she didn't need to lose weight and that this hypnosis business was hogwash'. So Ruth went back to being an overweight, subservient, angry, dismissed, devalued person in her own home.

Guilt

The Pleaser riddles you with guilt. It is constantly suggesting that you could do more for this person or that situation. It loves you to feel guilty, because it means that you will bend over backwards to please everybody even more. The Pleaser believes its opinion is right and will not let up until you meet its ransom. Guilt, I believe, is a wasted emotion. I know that we all feel guilt from time to time but the Pleaser loves hanging onto it to keep you looking after everybody else. It is a pure, unadulterated force of fearful concern. The fearful concern is one of being unloved and the result is often transferred to food.

Can you imagine having at your beck and call a 24-hour nursemaid who is sexually available all of the time as well as being a mother, cook, driver and social organiser? This is the Pleaser at its best.

The Pleaser, Affection and Sex

The Pleaser character trait loves being loved and, even more, loves giving love and therefore is often taken advantage of. The Pleaser personality may unconsciously look for a partner who represents the opposite to the Pleaser, so that they can continue to look after someone else's needs. An example of this is a Pleaser whose partner reflects the following type of behaviour: judgemental, critical and often selfish. The partner of a Pleaser enjoys the idea of having someone around who constantly looks after their needs.

Karen came to see me because she had recently met a guy who, in her words, 'was the one' and she was feeling out of control about how to handle the relationship. Karen said, "I worry about being attractive enough and good enough for him. I have always attracted men who have judged me on my weight and my looks. I've always felt I wasn't good enough. I always make sure I look good, I try and maintain a certain weight. I am always available for sex, whether it's been a long day or a lazy day. I feel exhausted trying to make my relationships work and yet they never last." Karen's relationship history was riddled with Pleaser character traits, not to mention low self esteem.

Karen had created an unconscious pattern of attracting men who kept her Pleaser on its tip-toes. Her desire for being loved was represented by how much she could look after 'her man' by being sexually available at any time. On a conscious level, she was horrified at how she responded to any sign of affection and, despite being horrified, she kept repeating this behaviour even though it was detrimental and did not result in a lasting relationship.

I am not suggesting that every Pleaser runs around having rampant sex but the bottom line is that Pleasers have the inability to say the word 'No', and this includes sex. Saying 'No' to sex is every individual's right, be they woman, man or child, and to say 'Yes' when you don't want to have sex does not lead to fulfilment. It is the Pleaser who says 'Yes' to the cake or biscuit your neighbour baked when you actually don't want to eat it. And it is the same Pleaser voice which says 'Yes' to food and sex just to please the other person.

On a more positive note, the Pleaser loves physical intimacy because the Pleaser loves giving and receiving love. Pleasers tend to be sensual people who love the taste and sensation of food and intimacy, for this is a way for the Pleaser to have its own needs met.

The trick is to keep the Pleaser in line with the Slim Confident part, so they are balanced and not undervalued. Through doing this, the Pleaser does not end up in emotionally vulnerable situations.

Track 2 will help you start to do this naturally. You will be ready to listen to this track after chapter 6.

The Inner Critic and the Pleaser

The explanation of Karen's self destroying behaviour can be taken even further. Her Inner Critic began voicing its opinion. Karen's Inner Critic was saying, "He thinks you're fat." while her Pleaser was saying, "You need love, do what he says because then he will love you." Her Inner Critic kept whispering, "You won't get anybody else. This is as good as it gets!" What chance did Karen have? She truly believed these statements made by her Inner Critic and her Pleaser.

The Inner Critic affirms your Pleaser traits by repeatedly saying, "You're so weak, you really need to sort this out, you don't even like that person - why did you say yes?"

There are many different reasons why weight loss can be difficult. However, losing the weight and maintaining the desired weight is a stumbling block for many, hence this book. Often a person's Inner Critic lives in fear of their Pleaser's desire to become intimate with someone else. This could, for example, be due to past sexual rejection or bad sexual experiences. A Pleaser person may also put on a considerable amount of weight to avoid intimate relationships. Their Inner Critic is so powerful that any sexual interaction would be too emotionally painful. The Inner Critic says, "Don't go there, you will just get criticised. Who wants to make love to a ball of blubber..." As the Inner Critic keeps going on and on, so to does the weight.

Anxiety, Food and Alcohol

The Pleaser says 'Yes' to every social invitation because they worry and become anxious they may offend if they say 'No'. This form of behaviour can be detrimental to your most important relationships, which include you.

You may recognise this Pleaser trait within yourself or perhaps you know of someone else who constantly runs around anxiously looking after other people. Now here is an interesting point: they don't do it because they like looking after other people - they do it to be liked. Of course we all like to help people from time to time, but the Pleaser creates anxiety within a person through doing too much. As a result, they run themselves ragged and deplete their energy by not saying 'No'.

Anxiety is a natural experience and is due most of the time to the Inner Critic's incessant chatter; however, the Pleaser is also a catalyst in the production of anxiety. That is why anxiety goes into overdrive in many people. The following is a typical situation where the Inner Critic steps into overdrive: it begins by replaying last night's dinner party where you entertained the parents of your child's new friend. Its voice tells you, "You could have done so much better. You could have been funnier. The beef was overcooked. The parents left a little too early. Perhaps you're not interesting enough." Then the Inner

Critic is joined by the Pleaser and together they run a check list through your mind. "Did I offend at any time? Maybe I could have said that or suggested this…" The list goes on, because the Pleaser is only concerned about you being liked and loved and not rejected. It's guaranteed that with these two on board you'll always feel there would have been something you could have done better.

The Pleaser's anxiety is primitively resolved by food and alcohol. The Pleaser bases itself on love, giving love and being loved. Pleasers tend to be squashy, cuddly people who are the life and soul of the party. They tend to be great cooks and are always organising fabulous dinner parties. They love food. It is a great cover up because they are achieving what the Pleaser wants. Number one on the list is that while they are nurturing their friends through food, they are also nurturing themselves.

After the dinner guests have left, the Pleaser, because of their love of food, will keep all the leftovers so they can feed themselves. And while they are doing this they play over and over again what they could have done better, funnier, kinder and so the list goes on. So what do these Pleasers do? They stuff their faces with food. Then what happens? They wake up in the morning with their Inner Critic going ballistic and their Pleaser saying, "They are going to reject you because of…"

Video Crazy

Pleasers are constantly complimenting other people and berating and belittling themselves. We talked about Radio Crazy before; however, this is even worse - it's called Video Crazy and this comes complete with visual effects of colour and movement together with voice! Video Crazy recall is over imaginative and completely effective in the way it works, and Stephen Spielberg would have a field day.

Pleasers press the remote control and replay the same scene over and over, and along the way the scene becomes embellished with imagined things. Unfortunately, the unconscious mind will believe the Video Crazy to be true, because the unconscious mind doesn't know the difference between reality and the imagination. The Video Crazy replay keeps reminding you of how much better you maybe could have acted. The role of pleasing can never be overdone.

Bullies

Pleasers have a sliding scale of who to look after first. The people who are the most difficult to please always come first. For example, Stacey had a bullying father who had an issue with her weight. He saw her physical imperfection as a sign of not being a successful father. Stacey's desperation for his approval led her to run around after him. She was in a blind panic, always trying to be the perfect daughter. She saw her mother as not a priority because her mother gave her unconditional love. She didn't need to appease her mother, and yet her mother deserved far more respect than her father ever did.

Bullies are only bullies because they get away with it. Underneath, they are frightened children. Pleasers live in fear of bullies and bullies live in fear of a Pleaser becoming confident and independent.

Pleasers' own problems

The Pleaser part is not keen on expressing how they feel about their life to other people. The Pleaser part finds this uncomfortable because it thinks that if people know that you are infallible, then you may not be there for them. Pleasers are always saying they are fine, and yet most of the time they are not. They are swimming in their own low self esteem because they do not value themselves as much as other people. This low self worth leads to moodiness and a sense of wanting to hibernate from the outside world. Pleasers need to retreat from time to time, simply to re-charge their batteries and sleep is a way of achieving this.

Ill Health

Pleasers don't often get sick but when they do, they do it well. Being ill is the only socially acceptable method of gaining attention. However, illness can lead to guilt. When a Pleaser is ill it means they cannot look after other people and this makes them feel guilty because they need taking care of instead of taking care of others. So they avoid getting ill at any cost. They also can be hypochondriacs sometimes, always having a worse disease than you.

Any illness is a concern; however, illness is also a safety mechanism to release the anxiety that the Pleaser has physically stored in the body. Being ill is also a method of being able to get away and rest from the anxiety - in other words, to have time out.

Mind Reader

The Pleaser part is often intuitive to other people's needs. It has trained itself to nurture and become a free therapist to the outside world. Like the Inner Critic, the Pleaser also thinks it can read other people's minds and to a certain extent it can. From time to time the Pleaser is quite intuitive because its role is to look after everybody else.

However, the Pleaser often gets irritated with the fact that people can't read their mind.

Inability to ask for help

An example of this was brought home to me by my relationship with my parents. I was a good child, always pleasing everybody else. I had loads of friends and was always busy, busy, busy, doing this or that. I was always tired and food seemed to be the only thing I allowed myself to experience. On one occasion a few years ago I asked my father, "Were you ever worried about me? Considering what you now know about how much I felt alone and unworthy as a person." He replied, "Georgia, I don't know how many times your mother and I wondered what was going on in that little mind of yours. You seemed happy most of the time, but when you used to retreat to your room we worried about what was going on and yet when we asked you how you were, you always responded with 'I'm fine.'" Yet I wasn't fine. I wanted my parents to take me away and tell me everything was all right and yet, as Pleaser, I didn't want to worry them. I overate because I felt different. I was too embarrassed to tell them this and yet I expected them when I got grumpy, depressed or upset to read my mind. I was in a no-win situation.

If you are a Pleaser, asking for help is generally a big issue. You are great at saying 'Yes' to everyone else, but opening up to your own problems and sharing them is unacceptable. Is it any wonder that after a while people stop asking you how you are, because you keep saying 'I'm fine'.

The Assertive Positive Pleaser

The Pleaser part has so much to offer you. It has a genuine desire for kindness, warmth, fairness and unconditional love that can be used for you too. It just takes practice.

If you look at all the qualities the Pleaser has to offer everybody else, you can see for yourself what a wonderful asset it can be. Imagine if you started to nurture yourself. At this point usually there is a little bit of uneasy stirring inside of you because the Pleaser is concerned that if you look after yourself then you will be rejected by other people. It is normal for a Pleaser to feel this way. I would be surprised if you didn't have any stirring. In fact if you don't have any stirring, congratulations - you don't have a strong Pleaser. Training your Pleaser to spend some time looking after you can be stressful and a little testing, to say the least, but the people you know will get used to it as you will, too. If someone doesn't like it, then the relationship clearly is not supportive and needed to change anyway. It's like starting a new relationship; however, this time it's with your self.

How the Pleaser can work with you rather than against you

The Pleaser is and always will be one of my strongest personality traits; however, now I use it to its positive advantage rather than its destructive use.

What a pleasure it is for me to still look after people but know it comes from my own choice rather than fear. I will always be a Pleaser and I like being a Pleaser. The Pleaser part of you means that you will always be interested in other people and the world around you.

Practice Privately

One of the best ways to introduce your assertive Pleaser part is to rehearse privately at home; for example, if you have a difficult relationship with your boss and perhaps you feel shy or unable to say what you want to say. Start to rehearse just a little something that you've been wanting to say to him for some time. Remember to take baby steps: this way you will gradually gain confidence. The best time to do this is while listening to the CD. While listening to the CD use all of your senses. What are you wearing? How are you sitting or standing? Feel your breathing supporting you to be confident. Remember, your unconscious mind doesn't know the difference between reality and imagination. So the repetition is simply going to affirm your library that pleasing yourself is a safe and normal experience. Perhaps at home, or somewhere where you can simply be with yourself, go over and over in your mind what you want to say in a kind but definite way. Other people say what they want to say. Why shouldn't you?

You have a choice

Being able to say what you want to say means that there is no mind reading going on. People are relieved when you say what you want because it makes it easier for them, not more difficult. It also means that you will be able to have healthier relationships with the people around you, and the beauty of this is that you will be able to achieve more because you have expressed to them what you want.

The alternative to not saying what you want is coming home angry that somebody else has had their way, but then of course there are always the chocolate biscuits to push your anger down with...

Being able to do what you want to do means you won't feel the need to push down your feelings with food, and you will feel more in control of your life. The domino effect of this experience is an increase in self esteem and healthier relationships with the people around you.

Embrace your Inner Pleaser as a wonderful part that now knows it is safe to be a little selfish with your time and your energy so that you can develop the self belief that will now enhance your life. Your world will blossom and so will you!

At the end of chapter 6, you will be ready to listen to track 2.

Chapter 5

The Perfectionist

What is the Perfectionist?

The Perfectionist is the part of us that has one very strict rule which you must abide by. And its rule is that you must achieve 100%, and if you can't achieve 100% then the Perfectionist tells you that you are a failure.

So often people say to me, "I am not a Perfectionist" and yet there will be an area of their life that is totally driven by their Perfectionist part. This could be achieving a high pass in an exam or perhaps running in and finishing a marathon. There is a lot of power and determination behind the Perfectionist, which is a good thing because it makes sure we apply ourselves diligently to what we undertake: however, there is also a down side to the Perfectionist which can be to the detriment of our self worth and confidence, and this can cause us problems.

The Perfectionist chapter is probably the hardest of all the parts for me to write about as its emotional presence in my life has not been as strong as for many of my clients. Often a strong Perfectionist trait will override the Pleaser personality; alternatively, if you have a strong Pleaser part, then the Perfectionist will not be as powerful. However, it has been my experience that both these parts are present when it comes to weight and food issues.

Busy People

Clare came to see me for a private consultation - she had two young daughters and was a full time partner in a prestigious law firm. Clare was running a very tight ship. She had heard about my work through a colleague who came to see me to stop smoking. Her colleague had given her a copy of my CD for relaxation. An immaculately well-groomed woman, Clare appeared to thrive on stress and the precision that it takes to keep everything perfect. When I asked Clare how I could help her, her response was that she wanted to lose some weight. I never assume anything prior to meeting my clients, and often do not know in advance why they made an appointment with me. Clare, like many of my clients, did not appear to need to lose weight. Weight, as you are aware, often is all in the mind. Sometimes it is an issue of small weight loss or perhaps bulimia. Emotional overweight does not necessarily represent itself physically. Clare's issue was just as real as the next person's.

Clare mentioned that she wanted to lose five pounds and you may as you read this think, "Five pounds? What is the point? After all, what is five pounds in the grand scheme of things?" Ironically, as it happened, at the time of Clare's appointment I felt like I had gained five pounds after a two week holiday in France: fortunately I knew how and why this had happened.

Clare then told me that she could not function properly unless she could get into her Versace jeans. They were her measurement of having lost or gained that infamous, illusive five pounds. The pattern of one month in Versace and the next not being able to do the top button up was driving her crazy. Clare lived a life of constant berating that she couldn't perfect that mysterious permanent weight of 8 stone 5lbs. I discovered that Clare was a binge eater and maintaining her perfect lifestyle to the outside world was causing her undue stress. In fact, it was her Perfectionist part that had been controlling her life, making sure that everything was perfect and in place. Clare's frustration was that all areas of her life were perfect. Great husband, two gorgeous children, nice house, great family and friends, and yet this one area, the elusive 8 stone 5lbs part of her life, she just could not get right.

Clare said, "By the time I can get into my Versace jeans they're going to be out of date. I am so bored of my constant thinking about those bloody Versace jeans. I spend more time thinking about my weight than I do about my work or my family. Sometimes I feel like I am going mad."

Of course Clare's Inner Critic was berating her and behind the Inner Critic there was a Perfectionist. Clare's Perfectionist managed all the other parts of her life extremely well, and yet Clare couldn't quite get the weight/bingeing sorted out.

The Perfectionist perfects not losing weight

Now at first the following concept may seem odd to you, but if you are either on a diet or losing weight it simply means your

Perfectionist has perfected bingeing and yo-yo dieting. The result is the unconscious mind thinks this is normal because it equates stress with overeating and anxiety with bingeing. Then the Inner Critic steps in and criticises the weight gain and the dieting cycle begins. So the Perfectionist equals overeating and the Inner Critic dieting and so the cycle goes on and on.

The Perfectionist unconsciously brings in all your past experiences of how to deal with negative emotions and says to you, "Where's the food?" and before you can blink you find yourself raiding the fridge. It is a practice that has been perfected over and over again. This form of overeating has been perfected to such an extent that any conscious recognition of this repetitive behaviour will be overridden because the Perfectionist part has you trained to overeat to perfection. Remember, the Perfectionist's job is to do things 100%, and Clare's conscious mind could not understand why this was happening and the consequence of this led her to more frustration and binge eating.

The Perfectionist Creation

Clare grew up in a family where life was always unpredictable. Clare's parents were in the music business. Home life was fraught and unpredictable with an assortment of people constantly moving in and out of the house, which was always messy. Her parents were hippy types who took each day as it came. This sort of lifestyle didn't suit Clare, so her unconscious mind made the decision that being a professional person was a much more reliable emotional state. You see, Clare liked predictability and being prepared, so she applied the

Good Girl Guide approach to life. For Clare, being prepared meant no surprises, or at least that was the plan. So Clare set about creating her daily life systems: this meant situations that she could perfect such as reliability - her plan was there would be no chaos in her life. There would be only balance in her life.

Setting Goals

We all have a Perfectionist to some extent, whether it is making sure we look nice for the Christmas party or making sure we plan the dinner party menu. Having a Perfectionist drive is healthy. The problem is that some goals the Perfectionist sets are unrealistic and even if we achieve these goals we sometimes find out they are not sustainable.

In the case of Clare and her Versace jeans, Clare had not taken into account life experiences. Stress is a normal part of everyday life. How we deal with it is an unconscious habit and it is this habitual aspect which is this book's focus. We all have situations in life that crop up which are beyond our control. Perfectionists have a problem with this, because it upsets their plan. The example of losing weight where the Perfectionist has set out with the best made plans to eat only fruit all day can be destroyed in an instant by an unplanned external situation.

There were many times in the past when I set out rules for myself to lose weight. All would be well until I was disrupted by a well-meaning friend who said, "Let's go out and have some fun." Being a Pleaser of course meant I had to say 'Yes' and then my attempt at losing weight was a failure and so I would binge for the rest of the week till Monday!

My Perfectionist knew just where to find the food. It had perfected disruption.

The Perfectionist, Holidays and Weddings

How often we read an article about a bride standing proud with 'before' and 'after' shots of her weight loss for her big day. What a wonderful goal to aim for, to feel fabulous on your wedding day. However, how many brides put the weight back on after the honeymoon period is over? Anybody who has been in this situation: please don't worry! You've just experienced another Inner Critic attack. The Perfectionist is great when there is a clear goal in sight or a deadline to work to, but what happens when the deadline is gone and the goal has been achieved?

Felicity has one month till her holiday, so she decides she would love to lose 10lbs so she can feel confident wearing her bikini. In her mind, a month is enough time to lose the 10lbs and she has read about the latest low carb, high protein diet in her favourite weekly magazine, so she sets her weight loss goal to be achieved by this eating regime. Felicity looks at her calendar to check her social engagements. In Felicity's mind, the only way she can successfully lose weight is not to go out, because by doing this she won't be tempted by wining and dining. A lot of people follow this common routine. So Felicity makes the decision that under no circumstances will she participate in any social activities. Now the reason for following this routine is actually to avoid an Inner Critic attack. Felicity, of course, is not consciously aware of this routine but deep down she knows that if she goes out and has a glass or two of wine her diet will go out the window and she will eat everything in sight.

All or Nothing

The Perfectionist has a real issue with the grey area of life. It thinks of everything as either black or white and there is no in between. The Perfectionist relationship within a person can often drive that person to extreme lengths to achieve their weight loss goals and, for that matter, any goals they may set.

In the case of dieting the Inner Critic loves it when Felicity goes into the grey area, the area of wining and dining, because it can start to voice itself, making such statements as, "Go on, have another glass of wine!" and "One more piece of chicken isn't going to hurt. You've blown it now - you may as well eat the rest of the chocolate. See? I told you, you're so weak." And so it goes on - the list is endless.

By avoiding these social tests and Inner Critic attacks Felicity can maintain her Perfectionist weight loss regime. Unfortunately, by following this common routine, Felicity has created for herself a mountain of anxiety.

The Inner Critic and its relationship with Success

In order to achieve weight loss you need to remember that the mind remembers every time you have lost and gained weight. It has memories of every successful time and every binge experience. The Inner Critic is part of your memory system, therefore every time you want to lose weight it will stir up every example of limited success and failure just in case you fail. The Inner Critic, as I have said, is there to protect you. It has travelled with and experienced your great highs and lows when it comes to losing weight, and the Inner Critic's main goal is to help you avoid being vulnerable. It has also felt the pain of your weight gain. The Inner Critic has also experienced the lack of self worth with binge eating and more importantly it has stored all these vulnerable times in its library. So it says, "Don't go there again – it's all too hard, it hurts too much." The Inner Critic tries to sabotage you before you do it to yourself. It is a shield that will at any cost make sure you are safe, but of course from the Inner Critic chapter we know that it is just one voice and is not always right.

The drive of the Perfectionist

When it comes to losing weight, setting realistic goals is great. However, the Perfectionist often has a different opinion. Felicity, as mentioned before, thinks that losing weight represents 100% commitment. This means every recipe is by the book and every almond is counted. In order to achieve success, the Perfectionist must avoid any Inner Critic comments because it will lead to the Complete Fall Off The Wagon Syndrome. So while Felicity is measuring every 100 grams of rice she knows she is on track. The energy it takes to stay on track is momentous. Just think about the sudden change in Felicity's lifestyle in order for the Perfectionist to achieve the weight loss goal.

With her social events completely out for a month, this means Felicity is under social and emotional restrictions. This leads to isolation, loneliness, feeling ostracised and, worse still, makes Felicity feel even more overweight than she really is.

The restriction of food means that she is thinking about food more than she would normally. Her mind monitors what she can and can't have to eat and drink. This then leads to cravings. We all know what we can't have, we want and the Inner Critic loves this stirring internal banter. Let's say, for example, that Felicity's Perfectionist has won for these four weeks and she has lost loads of weight and is feeling on top of the world. She is looking forward to her holiday and her spirits are high.

Felicity goes on her holiday without her Perfectionist: she has left it behind. Remember the Perfectionist is 100% there or not at all. Felicity has a fantastic holiday and comes back having gained a little of the weight she lost. She feels fine with this because she tells herself she will go back to what she was doing before, in moderation. 'In moderation' I say. The Perfectionist does not know moderation - it only knows all or nothing and so Felicity will start the same ritual all over again of losing and gaining weight.

Perfectionist traits lead to binge eating

This pattern of behaviour is extremely common. Whether it is trying to get into Versace jeans or going on that holiday, the underlying principle is the same. If you have a strong Perfectionist trait, when you are not dieting you will be binge eating.

I read once recently in a newspaper about the new terminology relating to emotional eating called 'permirexia' where someone is either on a diet or overeating. There is no in between. I see this in my work all the time. How much energy it must take for a person to maintain such diverse emotional states, and how much inner emotional turmoil is placed on that person to keep these two states going.

Perfectionists and Depression

If you have a strong Perfectionist part you may suffer from bouts of depression. If you are a high achiever and cannot accept coming second, or you do not get into a particular university, or perhaps you did not get a particular job or the relationship you 100% tried for, then it's guaranteed this will lead to an Inner Critic attack. And this leads to the knock-on effect which leads to the slippery slope of self loathing, anger, out of control feelings and binge eating.

Depression, I believe, is a natural emotional experience which we all go through from time to time and it is a sign that something is wrong in your life. I am not suggesting that anti-depressants should not be taken, but in many cases depression is the reaction to situations where there is a strong Perfectionist and/or Inner Critic dialogue going on.

You may perceive that external people and situations are demanding results from you, and if you have low self esteem you may take these demands too seriously and hide behind a strong Perfectionist. You then place yourself in the combination of Perfectionist and Inner Critic, and this is a sure-fire way to set yourself up for burnout and then depression.

Failure is simply not an option for a strong Perfectionist personality, so if it does occur the consequences can be frightening for the individual and the people around.

The Grumpy Perfectionist

I don't know how many Perfectionist people you know, but they can be very difficult people to work and live with. I admire people who are goal driven and Perfectionist: once they have their mind set on something you know that they will achieve it which is great, particularly if it is something you know is not your strength. The down side is that as the Perfectionists tend to suffer bouts of depression they can get snappy and have very heavy energy when they are in a down phase. This can often be jealousy at other people achieving what they wanted to achieve, or not having what someone else has which they want, and this includes weight loss.

The Perfectionist Perfecting Life

We know why magazine covers sell us the latest diet: because the 'dieter' within us all will go out and buy that magazine simply because a celebrity achieved weight loss through this or that particular eating regime. We are all looking for the perfect body. Perhaps you may have a friend who has lost weight through some form of eating programme. Your Slim Confident part is driven to suss the eating programme out, and the Perfectionist within us all is supporting this behaviour by perfecting the desire.

In my past when my diet went pear-shaped (no pun intended) I would become disgruntled, angry and retreat into myself. I would feel angry with the rest of the world including my closest friends, who in my mind didn't have weight and food issues. I would smile to the outside world and go to bed thinking how unfair my life was. My skinny friends had no idea of the pain I was going through. It was okay to talk about dieting but in my teenage years there was no awareness of bulimia and anorexia. People continue to suffer in silence because their Perfectionist part and their Inner Critic don't want to expose to the outside world, "What a mess you are in!" So to the outside world you look like you handle life perfectly.

I have a wooden plaque on my bathroom wall of a woman praying, saying desperately, "Dear Lord if you can't make me skinny can you please make my friends fat!" Now isn't that the truth! Deep down we are always looking at other people, what weight they are, what they are wearing and how they manage their lives. We measure our perfectionism on other people who have nothing to do with us. If it was that simple, my prayers would have been answered a long time ago and so would yours.

Maintaining weight equals anxiety

The Perfectionist can learn, from past failures at losing and maintaining a healthy weight, that even contemplating losing weight signals a no-go area. The Perfectionist only wants you to succeed, therefore it will protect you and lead to the art of gaining weight.

Karen from Belfast came on a two day workshop a few months ago. She was very vocal throughout the first morning. Karen debated with me suggesting that she was very good at losing weight. She just couldn't keep it off. I asked her how many times over her lifetime had she been successful at losing the weight and she replied, somewhat embarrassed, "My wedding, holidays, other people's weddings, you name it." Karen was clearly, as she said, 'very good at losing weight' but maintaining her goal weight was a real mystery to her. The fact was, somewhere within Karen's mind when she reached her goal weight, she was fine; however, maintaining it brought anxiety. This anxiety could have been triggered by any number of things, from her being noticed more or maybe it was because losing weight meant having to get on in life.

Is this it?

I can't tell you how many times clients have said to me that they thought their life would improve simply because they had lost the weight they wanted to. Apart from an increase in self confidence, which is fantastic, once they have reached their desired weight they notice the 'is this it?' syndrome going on. Apart from feeling physically fantastic, the idea that losing weight solves all your problems is simply not true. Yes, it does hopefully restore your body image and self esteem, but apart from that you've still got to work, sleep and socialise. The world around hasn't changed: people are still doing exactly what they were doing before. It is you who has changed and this can bring on anxiety itself.

Procrastination

When I lost a lot of weight, I felt fantastic, people commented on how brilliant I looked and the world seemed less stressful. After I had maintained the weight for a period of time, I realised that my life really hadn't changed. I had spent so many times in my life thinking, planning and dreaming about all the things I would do once I was slim that by the time I got there I had no excuses.

I had procrastinated most of my overweight life about everything, including losing weight. When I lost the weight I realised how much time I had spent saying, "I'll do it when I am slim. I won't be any good at it unless I'm slim. I won't book that holiday until I'm slim. I'll do that course when I feel more confident in myself." When I had lost the weight I found that I was feeling scared. I had no more excuses and anxiety set in. Of course, this triggered a slow but guaranteed weight gain and then I had another excuse: "I'll do it when I lose the six pounds I've just put on."

I had perfected keeping the weight on as it was the only way I could avoid getting on with my life. I see this often in my clinic world. A classic example of this is a client called Patricia, who I have been treating for binge eating. The first few weeks she was doing really well and feeling on top of the world. On the third appointment she came in crying because she had been bingeing all week. I asked her what had gone on that week, what was different to the previous two weeks and Patricia responded that nothing out of the ordinary had happened and that she had no idea why she had binged.

Binge eating only occurs when there is a preceding emotional trigger. No one binges simply because it just happens. There is always a trigger prior to the behaviour. So I knew in my heart that something was going on and that Patricia was not consciously aware of it.

On the fourth appointment, Patricia came back very disillusioned. She couldn't understand why the first two weeks went so well and now it was all going down hill. And then it happened! Patricia said she had come to see me to lose weight for a very special reason. She was due to have a breast reduction operation the next month and she was panicking that she wouldn't be slim to match her new smaller breasts.

Patricia had procrastinated all of her overweight life. While her breasts were a double F there was no point in losing weight. Her image of herself was that people only ever saw her breasts and that the rest of her body was never really in view.

To Patricia, having small breasts meant she had to get on with her life and lose weight. It was emotionally terrifying. No wonder she was binge eating. By training Patricia to feel safe losing weight, she perfected excitement at the prospect of her new breasts and body. She deserved to feel good about herself as everybody does. Patricia went through with her operation. She feels and looks fantastic!

Perfecting not being perfect is a great way to avoid life and the Perfectionist, when it comes to losing weight, will train itself to do just that. Perfecting not losing weight leads to more anxiety and out of control feelings.

The Perfectionist perfecting looking after the Slim Confident part

The all or nothing dieting syndrome, as mentioned earlier in this chapter, represents the Perfectionist being absolutely perfect at either losing or gaining weight.

The aim for you is to work with your Perfectionist rules so they work with you rather than against your best made plans. By listening to track 2 on the self hypnosis CD you can educate your mind that each week is not about being perfect. It's about perfecting having a good week. It may seem a little hard to imagine, but if the Perfectionist is educated to think that perfecting balance, logic and having self esteem is normal, then anxiety around food will start to lose its energy. It is once again about training the unconscious mind to see that life is a much safer experience and this means emotionally you're not reaching for food.

I can't express enough how important this process is. It is a valuable tool that can be utilised for any aspect of life. It's just not about losing weight. In fact, you may have noticed by now that the emotional tools you are learning are helping you in many other aspects of your life. That is what is great about hypnosis. It has a domino effect, such as sleeping better, feeling more positive and communicating more confidently.

If you read every article written about my work you would notice a common theme. It's about training the mind to perfect responding to life positively through good times, boring times, stressful and fun times. It's about trusting in the flow of life and that life is very rarely perfect.

Let's face it, there is always going to be another business lunch, a party, a family outing. This is life and nobody should be expected to have to retreat into a hole while they are trying to lose weight.

By training your mind to simply trust that each week represents a good week, rather than perfect, the pressure is off you to lose weight successfully 100% every second of the day and night. It is simply not possible to maintain such Perfectionist demands because life just isn't like that.

By listening to track 2 after the next chapter, you will notice that perfecting having a good week is becoming more comfortable for your Perfectionist. It's about perfecting balance, being rational, patient and kind from you to you.

Chapter 6

Inner Child

What is the Inner Child?

Every time I work with the Inner Child of my clients, and in fact my own Inner Child, I always experience a melting pot of different emotions, the most powerful emotion being vulnerability. The Inner Child is pure unadulterated vulnerability and is a major player in the Inner Dialogue approach.

The Inner Child is the part within us all that loves to play, cry, be touched and loved. It is the raw emotional state that can hold us back in our adult world, simply because our Inner Child has been suppressed in the process of us developing into adulthood. If you had to grow up internally before your natural childhood age or perhaps grew up in a family where affection was scorned, your Inner Child will have learned very quickly that asking for love and affection will only get you into trouble. When the Inner Child becomes frightened it hides away deep within the unconscious mind, often only appearing at certain times as demonstrated through this chapter.

The Inner Child is a wonderful loving part within all of us. The great thing about exploring your relationship with your Inner Child is that it can lead you to a much deeper and more powerful knowing about who you really are. Spending time with this part means you become more whole in your outlook of yourself and the relationships around you.

The Inner Child part only knows how to be and it expresses itself in many different ways. The following questions are examples of the many different emotional facets to the Inner Child.

- When was the last time you had a real belly ache laugh?
- When was the last time you had a really good cry?
- When was the last time you wanted to be stupid?
- How often do you rebel like a naughty child?
- When was the last time you enjoyed being loved?
- Do you feel safe in intimate situations?
- Do you often feel isolated from people with a sense of loneliness?
- Do you often feel sad?
- Is anger something that you find hard to express?
- Do you find anger is overused in your life?
- Are you frightened of being out of control?
- Do you get annoyed when people are being silly?
- Do you drink to add fun to your life?
- When you drink alcohol do you become angry?

All of the questions above relate to the different emotions that the Inner Child within all of us experiences from time to time.

Childhood

The Inner Child is the child-like part of us that has never grown up, and it is the part within that should never grow up for its sole purpose is keep us in touch with our unprocessed emotions.

I was walking through Hyde Park in London the other day and sat for a few moments observing the world around me. There was the most beautiful little girl with her father, playing together, totally absorbed in each other. Watching them together brought tears to my eyes as the little girl's total trust, innocence and unconditional love towards her father was so obvious. It was such a magical moment in my mind and also appropriate considering I was in the middle of writing this chapter. This child was having so much fun and her father was, too, and I smiled thinking wouldn't the world be a better place if all children could experience the moment I had just witnessed? Unfortunately, we all know this is not the case for everyone and the truth is the little girl I saw with her father may not have the opportunity to be a child for long, for this will depend on her upbringing.

Becoming More Adult

Mark came to see me about his inability to commit to a relationship. Mark had come from a traditional family where his mother stayed home and his father was the breadwinner. Mark's family led a fairly insular life. He said he couldn't recall much socialising and his parents never really argued, his mother just always agreed with what his father said. He recalls affection was not common between any of the family. When he was 10, he discovered his father was having an affair.

Mark didn't fully understand what this meant, except that his father moved out of his parents' house and he and his brother were told not to ask questions. It was all very hush-hush at the time. His mother told Mark that he would need to grow up fast so he could become the man of the family and he did just that. Mark's unconditional love for his mother and seeing how hurt and frightened she was meant his needs took second place. Because of this, Mark's Inner Child was immediately suppressed and overnight his childhood became a thing of the past.

Alcohol

In the adult world Mark had shied away from serious relationships. Every time he got too close, he would break off the relationship. Mark was 32 at the time he came to see me in the clinic, and he was desperate to sort this situation out. He was drinking way too much and had put on a lot of weight. He said he had got into a habit of having a few too many beers after work and that any sexual encounters involved consumption of alcohol before he could even contemplate intimacy. Mark had trained himself to become so adult that his Inner Child only came out when he drank.

Alcohol, for a lot of people, is a way for their Inner Child to come out and play. So how many people drink to bring their Inner Child out? Probably most people and that is OK; however, when it has become a health issue as well as a method to become more whole, then more serious problems occur.

Mark's problem was not so much the alcohol but the emotional stirring that occurred prior to drinking. Alcohol was the symptom, not the cause, of his heavy drinking.

Our Inner Child never goes away no matter how old we are, but it can become suppressed through life experiences, so much so that we feel it has gone away and left us until we drink and then it releases itself. How often do you see people who are quite serious by nature after a few drinks become so much nicer, softer and kinder?

The Inner Critic and the Inner Child

The Inner Critic can sometimes be suppressed when we drink and this results in us becoming funnier, more out-going and taking more risks. We can become silly and people who don't normally cry may experience tears during this time. We don't care that much about the consequences until we wake in the morning and have a massive Inner Critic attack. The Inner Critic says, "You were such an idiot last night, what did you think you were doing? Everybody is going to laugh at you when you go into work on Monday. People are going to think you're screwed up because you couldn't stop crying." The list goes on and on, but the fact is the Inner Child felt safe to come out and play because the Inner Critic had gone away.

Responsibility

The Inner Child doesn't know what responsibility is, it just knows how to be and in the adult world being responsible means shutting down the Inner Child part. Adult behaviour means good work ethics, social standing and not rocking the boat. Who wants to be serious and responsible all the time? Well, that is how a lot of people were brought up.

A child who has experienced sexual, physical or emotional abuse will learn very quickly that remaining a child only exacerbates more abuse, therefore shutting down this innocent, wide-eyed, beautiful part is the best method of protection. To these adults being a child signals hurt, abandonment and abuse, so their Inner Child digs itself deep inside the mind. Why would you want to remain a child if this is what represents childhood memories?

Family Dynamics

One of my clients, Felicity, came to see me about her weight. Felicity was 5 stone overweight at the time. Felicity's father was an alcoholic and when he was drunk he would regularly beat her mother and verbally abuse her and her two sisters. Felicity found solace in food, and from her teenage years started to gain a lot of weight. She also started standing up to her father and protecting her mother. We discussed whether Felicity had unconsciously chosen to put weight on to become big and strong to protect her mother and siblings. She thought perhaps this was the case, but aside from this it was clear to me that her family life played a major part in her relationship with food.

We will never have the perfect family life, it just doesn't happen; however, what we do know is that most parents do the best they think they can at the time, even if it wasn't in your opinion good enough. All types of people become parents and their map of life doesn't necessarily need to become yours.

Fear of Intimacy

Mark had a fear of intimacy. The only way he could express his loving side was after a few beers, when his Inner Child became free to express itself. His adult part would have said, "Don't go there - to be open with your affection is not right."

Gaining weight can be a great way of suppressing our sexual side because perhaps we don't feel we deserve to be loved. The Inner Child loves hugs and kisses. If being sexual is an unsafe place to be, then gaining weight can be a way to alleviate the anxiety or fear of rejection.

Intimacy is a wonderful expression of our true selves. It is our right as adults to be able to express physical love. With Mark, it was a matter of training his Inner Child to know it was safe to come out without the use of alcohol. The aim wasn't for Mark to become the joker or the Agent 007 of the office, but rather to embrace his right to express himself safely while sober. Free in his knowledge that it was safe for him to express his Inner Child meant Mark cut back on his alcohol consumption, he was losing weight and the people around him started to notice how much calmer and more confident he was. Not only was the hypnosis helping him to re-connect to his own Inner Child, but he was also becoming much more relaxed about his life. Freeing this lovely gentle part of Mark meant he became more playful and happier, therefore he smiled more. Coincidentally I saw Mark in an office block reception area recently - our eyes connected and he smiled at me and patted his flat stomach.

Anger and the Inner Child

Anger is a big one when it comes to suppression of the Inner Child, for anger is a major player in the expression of a hurt, wounded child. Once again, when alcohol is consumed, the angry Inner Child can come out and be spiteful, hurtful and abusive just like Felicity's father.

Bullying tactics are often based on a wounded child. Better to become the bully rather than the victim. I do truly believe that no-one deep down wants to hurt anyone - it is simply a protective mechanism to avoid vulnerability.

A wounded child can resort to alcohol, food, drugs and abusive relationships simply because this is the only way the Inner Child knows how to be. It is sad but true: there are many wounded inner children walking around in adults, just waiting to express their anger and this anger plays a major role in expressing the hurt and rejection these adults felt during their childhood.

Just to recap chapter 3 again, each of us early on while growing up created emotional habits to enable us to get on in life. Each of these habits, at the time, was an emotional reflex action with limited knowledge of the world around us. Remember: food, love, tears and laughter are the first learned experiences. No wonder so many of us see food as a way to nurture ourselves. The surprise is when we get to adulthood we try and shake off these primitive habits and that is where the frustration starts. Consciously you think to yourself, "Why can't I just eat normally like other people do? What's wrong with me? I want to lose weight like other people do. Why can't I just have one piece of toast, not four?" The Inner Child has learned to express itself through food and plenty of it. Food is a way to stuff down fear, anger and abandonment.

Children don't understand 'No'

The Inner Child within all of us is open to exploring new experiences and loves new and exciting things. As we know, children get bored very easily and entertainment is high on the agenda: just ask any parent. When a child is told 'No' the immediate reaction is to rebel. The child does not understand that 'No' means 'absolutely not'. A child does not have the capacity to comprehend all the rules of adult life and nor should it, therefore people who struggle with their weight may have this rebellious streak in them, therefore they rebel against 'No'.

I remember when I was 14 having a crush on one of my sister's boyfriend's friends. I worked part time in the local late night supermarket. This boy used to pick me up from work to drive me home and I would pretend he was my boyfriend. One night my family and friends were sitting around watching a movie. I had bought loads of chocolate for everyone to share. I bent over to reach for my 25th piece of chocolate, only to be told by my heart throb that I couldn't afford to eat that much chocolate. I snapped back saying I'd paid for it and I could afford it. He remarked, "Yes, but Georgia - can you really afford to eat that chocolate?" I was so upset. I remember feeling so embarrassed at his comments that I decided, or should I say my Inner Critic decided, that I was obviously fat and unattractive so why not just keep eating and getting fatter? My Inner Child was so wounded that the easiest answer was to overeat. Nothing else seemed to alleviate the pain of rejection like food did.

The Inner Child and Bulimia

The Inner Child needs to understand that there are so many other ways of being heard rather than by food. Of all of the parts, the Inner Child can often be the most stubborn when it comes to letting go of binge eating as it does fulfil a primitive child-like desire. Re-parenting your Inner Child may seem a little scary at first, particularly as he/she does not like change.

Kathleen, a workshop participant, was well aware of her Inner Critic and was enjoying getting to know her Inner Dialogue; however, when it came to dealing with her Inner Child she really struggled. Every time she tried to listen to the Inner Child CD track she felt sick. She had this incredible urge to leave the course after the Inner Child section. Fortunately she came back the next week and reported to me and the group that her Inner Child had completely rebelled and she had been binge eating and vomiting all week. She felt disappointed that she had let herself and the group down (a Pleaser trait).

Bulimia is very common with wounded inner children. The child is ravenous and the adult is reprimanding. There is this desire to eat absolutely everything in order to stuff down anger or hurt, you name it, then the Inner Critic kicks in and the panic begins. I personally have never been bulimic, I tried but chickened out.... but the pain I hear expressed from my clients makes me feel like I have been there myself.

The problem for Kathleen was as her Slim Confident part was developing, her Inner Child began to panic because food was her only known resource to get attention. I asked Kathleen to go home and write down all the fears that her Inner Child had. I asked her to sit quietly and dialogue with her little Kathleen. She broke down and cried and this is what she said: "I don't have any images of little Kathleen. I don't think she has ever been there. She is lost amongst all this fat. I can't stand this pain. It hurts so much. Food seems to be the only way to ease it." It was a powerful scene and the group kindly wrapped her with lots of hugs and love. She was in floods of tears by this stage and I was just holding myself together.

I asked all of the participants if they would mind if we did some more Inner Child work as a group and they all kindly agreed.

I wrote down on the board all of the things that the group would have wanted for their own Inner Child had they had the opportunity and the list they voiced went on and on. One participant piped up with: "I always wanted a dog, but because my parents travelled so much and I was at boarding school I was never given that opportunity." Kathleen's face completely changed. She recalled her parents had decided that when she was 7 years of age she would go to boarding school. Kathleen had a dog called Woofa and they were inseparable. Little Kathleen was inconsolable having to leave Woofa to go to boarding school. The first school break she arrived home to find out that Woofa had been taken away to live on a farm. No one told Kathleen and she was devastated that she never had the chance to say goodbye. Kathleen went back to boarding school feeling lost, abandoned and emotionally disconnected to her parents. The only unconditional love she had received was from Woofa. The rest of the group was crying as Kathleen told her Woofa story and when Kathleen finished she felt a penny had dropped. She knew from that moment that she had buried her memories of herself as a child, because Woofa was in every picture.

Kathleen no longer felt nausea. It was like the weight literally had been lifted from her mind. Kathleen learnt to see herself with Woofa again through her own inner parenting skills, and during the process she lost her aversion to dogs, too.

The Confident Fun Inner Child

How wonderful it is to see a child who is allowed to embrace their childhood fully. The confident child who is allowed to be naughty while being safely cautioned and guided through unconditional love. A child who is allowed to speak up and encouraged to be heard. A child who is allowed to play and have wildly creative thoughts. I love to hear their delightful laughter and see the beauty in the smiles on their faces.

If you feel this was not part of your childhood you can embrace these experiences as an adult. It does take practice but the lovely thing is, it is accessible. Re-learning through your inner parent's eyes, not the parents you had but your own ideas of parenting, therefore enabling you to bring out your own confident fun child-like part.

Here are some exercises that might help you explore your own Inner Child safely, so that you can spend more time with you and the innocent fun loving person you are and deserve to be.

Nature

Take a walk on your own to a place where you know you feel safe. Perhaps walking through a park, taking the time to sit and look at the beauty of nature. When we view nature through the eyes of the inquisitive child, we notice how much beauty there really is in this world. Notice the birds and the colours of the trees. If it is snowing, make a snowman or run through the autumn leaves.

The Movies

Rent out a really funny movie on your own or with someone you feel you can really be yourself with. Laugh like you want to laugh rather than suppressing it. Hire a movie that is a real tear jerker and have a fantastic cry all on your own. Laughing and crying are great ways of releasing tension, fears and anxieties of the Inner Child.

Writing

Write a letter to yourself explaining that you did the best job possible as a child with the resources that you had. Explain to her/him that now as an adult you are going to make sure that you and your Inner Child can safely express to each other any emotions of fear, rejection, abandonment and love.

Make a list of all the things you would love to do that you feel a little silly or shy about doing. An example of this could be joining an art or dancing class that you've always wanted to but felt too scared to try. Perhaps you could go to a pop concert that your adult part says you're too old to go to. You are never too old to have fun.

Imagination

As the unconscious mind doesn't know the difference between reality and imagination, find time to lie on your bed or sit in a chair, close your eyes and spend some time with your Inner Child. Do you have a clear image of yourself as a child? If not, look at a photograph or create an image in your mind that you feel best represents you as a child. Let your mind talk to him/her: tell your Inner Child they are now safe and you are available as the inner parent at any time to hear their call for help. Tell them that you are always there now no matter what happens, and that it is safe to be loved, to have fun and enjoy the wonders of life. I do warn you this can be a highly emotional experience. Be prepared for some tears. It can be a very cathartic experience and a well-deserved one. You have the right to embrace your Inner Child because no-one will ever be able to know your child the way you do. It is a very special relationship, a bond that will always be there. An Inner Child when nurtured will give you so much emotional support, laughter and lightness in your life and the best thing of all your Inner Child doesn't cost you anything!

My Inner Child

I remember when I left Australia to start life a new life, I was very scared. My Inner Child did not want to leave my parents, but my desire to find out who I was led me into this unknown northern hemisphere where I knew very few people. I remember when I locked myself into my seatbelt on the plane how scared I felt. I knew my little Georgia was seriously panicking. She was not happy at all with this move. Like all children she didn't understand why I had to do this, why couldn't I just stay in Australia where I had loving parents, sister, friends and a good quality of life?

I have very clear images of my childhood and fortunately they are lovely images. When I got onto that Qantas flight heading for California to train in Voice Dialogue, I sat little Georgia on my knee and I promised her I would never lose her. I told her that she was always safe with me and that I would always hear her whenever she needed me. I made that pact to myself and whenever I get frightened or scared I hold little Georgia so tight sometimes in my mind and heart I can't stop crying. My tears were reflecting her fears and lack of understanding as we travelled into another unknown realm of life. As I type this now I have tears flowing down my cheeks, as my little Georgia has the biggest smile ever and she completely trusts me now in whatever we do.

Children and their Aspirations

My mum has a brilliant Inner Child and when we get together we have so much fun, playing like children, laughing and crying safely. I often thank my mum for our special relationship. Her parents allowed my mum to really be a child for as long as she needed to 'be'. My grandmother, called Narnie, told me a lovely story about how mum always wanted to go to Hollywood. Mum wanted to be on the stage. She had dreams of being the next Betty Grable and being a very determined 6-year-old, mum told Narnie that she was going to take the next boat to Hollywood and that her mother wasn't going to stop her. My grandmother kindly looked in the phone book and suggested that she give the Port Authority a call to find out the boat times.

Mum excitedly asked the man who answered the phone, "Can you tell me the when the next boat to Hollywood is leaving?" The man on the end of the phone said, "Get off the phone, you silly little girl." Mum was devastated. She couldn't work out how the man knew she was a little girl and that he wasn't taking her seriously. My grandmother held her and said, "He just doesn't know children." The point is, children have dreams and they are often shattered by adults who have lost touch with this innocence. Children's dreams have no limitations. My mother was allowed to dream. Were you?

Final Note

I hope from this chapter that any emotional stirrings you have felt from time to time while reading now have a place in your heart and mind.

Child-like thoughts can often be irrational but also fun and full of life and energy. All of us have these wonderful inner children and now they have a home to go to. It is your gift from you to you. To be able to love, give love, to make love, to laugh and cry are each hidden treasures that are available to us all.

Enjoy your Inner Child because it is the only one you will ever really, truly know.

You can now enjoy listening to track 2.

Chapter 7

The Past, Present and Future

What is the Past?

The past is any experience that happened even one second ago. Every moment of our life experience is automatically stored within the unconscious mind.

The unconscious mind is not chronological. We know this for a fact, simply because if I asked you to remember something that happened five years ago, you would not have to scan back through the last five years. If you did go back literally each day of your life for the past five years you would be exhausted and not able to be in the present. You wouldn't move forward by re-experiencing the day to day life you have lived.

The unconscious mind has an amazing ability to use emotions to produce memories. If I asked you to recall your strongest memory of somebody commenting about your weight or your relationship with food, I could almost guarantee that it would still be as fresh in your mind as when it happened. It would also be interesting for you to note just how long ago that first experience was and how much it still triggers feelings of anxiety and rejection. Do you recall every second of the experience? Do you remember who said it? Of course you do. You remember what you were wearing and how you reacted. How did this moment affect you? Did it change your opinion about yourself?

The Filtering System

Memories are filtering into your mind every day as a reference to show you how to behave. It doesn't matter if they are from years gone by – it's irrelevant. The memories are there for a very good reason, to show you how to react and they do it in a millisecond.

When you experience a situation that you have experienced before, your mind doesn't need to create new information because it already has an example of how to react. If you don't have the information in your memory bank then automatically your mind will find something similar or create a new piece of information ready for the next time, so you know how to respond.

Memories are all you have to support your behaviour until you learn something new and that is why the CD is such an important part of this book, because that is where the new learning begins. I know I sound like a broken record but your mind does have the ability to create any thoughts and hypnosis is a great way to start.

Does this little girl's experience trigger your past?

I had the privilege of meeting a beautiful little girl called Emily, aged 7, who came to see me with her mother because she was being bullied at school. Children are wonderful hypnotic subjects because they are so open to learning. Emily's mother had been to see me the previous year, so she knew the work that I do and she thought I might be able to help Emily. I re-arranged my diary so that I could see her that week. The thought of a child being bullied horrifies me, so the sooner I could treat Emily, the better. Emily is from a half Chinese/white English family and her mother had briefed me on Emily's anxieties. She wasn't sleeping well and was crying, kicking and screaming that she didn't want to go to school.

When Emily and her mother arrived we sat down and had a chat. I explained what I do and the sort of things to expect during the hypnosis. I then asked her what was going on in her life that was upsetting her. Emily said to me that she dreaded every Tuesday because that was the day of her sports lesson and it meant that no-one would choose her. People who don't get picked for games are never good at sport. Nobody, it appears, likes somebody who isn't good at sport. Emily said she loved Tuesday evenings because she would feel relaxed for a few days, but by the weekend she was already dreading the build-up to the next Tuesday. I asked her if there was anybody in particular who she felt scared of. Emily said that one of the boys at school told her, "My mum said that Chinese people are skinny because they live on rice and vegetables. She says it's because they are poor - what happened to you?"

Emily is a typical naturally rounded child and to me she represented normal size. We know through our knowledge of child development that how the child is developing often has nothing to do with food issues. And this was so in Emily's case. My immediate concern was that if Emily believed she was overweight and bad at sport then it could become a self-fulfilling prophesy.

I asked Emily if she was chosen more often, would she like sport more? She said she didn't really enjoy it, although she loved skiing with her parents. I said, "Ah, so you are good at sport then?" She smiled. I recognised that Emily was displaying a classic confidence issue because her Inner Critic had raised its voice.

The aim of my hypnosis with Emily was to train her confident Inner Self to recognise that sport is a small part of the school week and that life has bits in it that we don't necessarily like, but that's OK and that she is OK. The CD I made for Emily reflected her confidence as a skier and how she could reflect this ability at school. If she could ski down a mountain then she was good at sport and nobody could deny that, not even her self. I explained to her mind that there can be a number of sports we don't like and there are some that we do and this is quite normal and natural. I wanted Emily to feel more relaxed about the sports lesson itself and that the more she was at ease with the fact it was simply just another lesson, the time would pass very quickly. So sports lessons would now equal feeling calm and confident.

Emily's mum phoned the next week to say that she was much brighter and that she listened to her CD every day. The weekend had been, for the first time, stress free and Emily had come home from school on Tuesday night and was very blasé about the sports lesson. Emily's mother also told me that Emily now wanted to go skiing more often.

Childhood Memories

School can be a stressful experience for so many children. Whoever created that old saying 'sticks and stones may break my bones but words will never hurt me' had it completely wrong. Words are the most powerful things of all and the boy's hurtful comment will be stored by Emily and, for that matter, by everyone who read it.

Memories can be the most powerful hindrance to anybody's progression from the present into the future. So many memories reflect old experiences that interrupt any natural desire to do something new or different. The sad thing is, most of these childhood memories are comments from external people, whether it was a school friend, family member or teacher. All external criticism is deeply absorbed and is always readily available to be recalled.

I know one of my first conscious memories of somebody commenting about my weight was when I was 13 years of age. I remember as clearly as I am sitting here now writing this book that I was standing in the school hall in my sports uniform with a group of friends. The sports teacher said in front of all of my peers, "Georgia, put your stomach in. What has happened to you, you used to be such a little thing." I was completely devastated and highly embarrassed. My friends were embarrassed for me, too; however, her destructive comment was cemented in my young mind and when nobody picked me as usual for the netball team that day I felt a complete failure.

People's opinion about other people's weight

I find it really sad that some people don't want to be associated with overweight people. It seems like a disease they are frightened they may catch. Interestingly, people have the same reaction when someone is made redundant from their work. Suddenly, without explanation, their friends drop away and phone calls are not returned and this leaves them feeling bewildered, hurt and alone. I pose this question: "How much of this type of behaviour by other people regarding weight and redundancy has to do with social status?" Most of us would like to be successful and popular people and being overweight, to some people, means that you may bring down their image to the outside world and therefore they avoid being seen with you.

If you have been rejected in the past because of your weight, please don't worry: you don't need those people in your life anyway! Just trust that you have the right to move on from the past and nobody can stop you from achieving this. Absolutely no-one! Through reading this book and listening to the CD you are building a library of the present and the future that will overlap your past. You are creating a safe haven for yourself so that anybody who tries to bring you down will not infect you with their ugly and contagious comments.

The Present

What I find fascinating is that we often think in the past or the future rather than the present. We are always aiming for something ahead in the future and this is natural; however, spending time in the present is a valuable emotional asset. To live now and enjoy this moment is an asset we need to appreciate.

My client base at The Wren Clinic, in the business district of London, is full of very stressed city workers mainly from the banking, insurance and legal industry. They come for a range of issues, from stopping smoking to insomnia. In fact, insomnia is a classic example for discussing the present, because not being able to sleep represents worrying about tomorrow or yesterday. It has nothing to do with the present.

I like to train my clients to be more in the present through understanding how to practise being in the present and not focus on what will happen next week or what happened last year which they have been doing 24 hours a day. We all need a break from constant measuring where we've been and where we are going. It is about learning to just be, being suspended in whatever you are doing and not worrying about the future or regressing back into the past.

Taking Time Out

Being in the moment does take practice, particularly if you have a strong Perfectionist. Pleasers tend to be better at it because they tend to love sleep as it is a way to retreat from the world. If you are aware that you don't take enough time out for yourself, try, even once a week, just sitting down and reading a magazine. Taking time out is invaluable for your mental wellbeing. Walking to clear your mind does the trick for a lot of people and it is inexpensive and beneficial for the body as well as the mind. As you are walking, notice what is around you rather than what is in your head. Listen to the sounds, be aware of the feel of your feet contacting what you are walking on, and absorb the different smells. If you stop for coffee, enjoy the taste. Get out of your head, enjoy the environment by being and doing in the moment, rather than focusing on the past or future. It does take practice but it will help your stress levels and clear your head.

For a lot of people, not focusing on the future all the time scares them and creates anxiety. These people feel they will lose the reins on their life if they don't keep on track. And so they look ahead constantly, working on the next project or the next job: the consequence is they take on too much and in doing this become seriously stressed. The truth is, trying to do too much creates burnout.

A lot of my clients tell me that when they go on holiday they come down with a cold. This happens because they haven't taken time out to be in the moment, to enjoy being in the present: as a result their minds have driven their bodies too fast and placed them under extreme stress trying to manage everything, so when they stop on holiday their bodies release all the tension through the illness. Holidays are an important aspect of all of our lives. Please, if you have the opportunity, don't feel guilty, and take the time out to enjoy being in the present. It is invaluable to the quality and length of your life.

One of the many bonuses of listening to the CD is that it is a wonderful way to achieve just being in the moment. While you are listening you can just drift away knowing that this is your special time out and you have chosen to experience being in the present. I also do talk about the future in the CD, but self hypnosis is about being in the present, about taking one moment at a time. It's about enjoying each day as a separate experience. It's a great stress management tool in itself.

The Jail Sentence of Losing Weight

One of the biggest hurdles my clients come across is that it takes time to lose weight. People get impatient because they want the weight off now, and they lose momentum because of the pure weeks and months it takes to lose weight. We measure everything in time slots such as birthdays, Christmas, holidays to mention a few. The whole idea of thinking about how much time it takes to lose weight can often put people off. The very thought of spending a whole year losing weight seems such hard work.

In traditional dieting terms it can be likened to a jail sentence, just like in the Perfectionist chapter. Traditional dieting means precision, concentration and, depending on how much weight you want to lose, six months of hard labour. Clients often say, "Well, it took me years to put it on, so of course it is going to take me a while to lose it." The point is yes, it may have taken years to put the weight on but it was done without much conscious effort. How often are we surprised to find all of a sudden that pair of jeans doesn't fit any more or that skirt is too tight? Weight goes on effortlessly and yet losing it seems to take a lifetime.

Taking each day as it comes

Being able to move on from the dieting mentality means a tension is released. No strict rules or regulations on what you should be doing, eating and drinking. The burden is lifted: you become free. There isn't the pressure to perfect a 100% successful weight loss week for it is about balance and that means taking one day at a time. It's about seeing each day as a new day separate from the last day and different to the next day.

Changing your relationship with food comes from increasing your confidence and motivation. It is about your Inner Dialogue working with your lifestyle: this is how you achieve a slimmer you instead of trying the myriad diets offered in the weekly magazines, then losing weight only to put it back on again. The Inner Critic loves these magazines because you keep measuring yourself against yourself on how much weight you should lose. Working with your eating routine and not somebody else's will make everything easier, and for some it does mean taking each day as it comes and enjoying it.

It's like slicing up the salami and seeing that the bigger picture is made up of little individual moments. They're your moments, not anybody else's. Each meal represents being in the moment so that you enjoy what you eat, letting go of any Inner Critic comments that represent your past or its fears for your future. Letting go of anxiety-producing comments such as, "Is this piece of cake going to make me fat?"

Every person on this planet earth is different, and taking one day at a time means that each week for you will be a great week because the one heavy-duty wining and dining experience does not spread its infection to any other day. It is simply living life.

When you stop berating yourself emotionally about what, when and how you eat you are free to enjoy life. Food isn't an issue any more and when food isn't an issue, you will not need to carry the weight emotionally and physically.

The Future

Most of the hypnosis work I do relates to moving on from the past, whether it is an anxiety disorder, lack of self belief or food/weight issues. The past is holding you back most of the time to the detriment of fulfilment of all of your hopes and dreams.

Perhaps you might like to ponder over what you envisage your future holds. This doesn't necessarily have to relate to your weight, but think about all the different things you would like to have or achieve.

Different Areas of your Future

I would like you to read through the next four sections with an open mind. Please leave your Inner Critic outside the door of your mind. If you feel any stirring of negativity remember, just like I mention on the CD, release it on the next breath out. Remember: any negativity you feel stirring is an old habit.

Personally

What would you like to do to enhance your life personally at the present moment? Perhaps you would like more confidence when socialising; maybe feel you would like to attract a new circle of friends. I want you to take your time and think about all the different opportunities that are out there in this big, wide, wonderful world for you to experience. Now write a list of everything that you have ever thought about doing, even if it seems totally outlandish. Remember, these are your thoughts and desires and as no-one else can read your mind, you are free to think of whatever you really want.

Professionally

A lot of my clients get stuck in a rut because they simply do not know what they want to do other than the work they are doing. I completely understand. I didn't know what I wanted to do till I was 28 either. If you are working, ask yourself: are you happy in your job? I know we all have to work to survive - that's life - but just for a moment think about a type of work that you feel really truly suits you. Be honest with yourself. Perhaps you have a sense of excitement when you think about the type of work you desire to do or a creative idea that has potential to be a business. Whatever it is, write it down, no matter how crazy the idea may seem.

Physically

Do you have a clear image of yourself becoming slimmer? Perhaps you have a photograph of a time in your life where you felt really good about yourself or, even better, you can create a future image of where you want to be physically. I want you to write down every aspect about the image that best represents the slim you.

Emotionally

Now I want you to look at the list under each area: personally, professionally and physically. Check in with yourself. What do you want to feel having achieved one or more of these experiences? Would you like to feel safe, excited, respected, supported or perhaps feel free?

Our desires to have a better life are always there and it doesn't necessarily come in the form of money, either. I want you to really study the list of your life goals. Notice any stirring inside which could be the voice of your Inner Child who is happy, or perhaps the Perfectionist who tells you that you won't be able to do it because you will have to do it 100% perfectly. The Pleaser also may not like it, because you are looking after yourself for a change. Enter into a dialogue with these parts, explaining that it is safe now for you to achieve these experiences. Keep dialoguing: soon they will get used to you doing this. The good news is that your inner Slim Confident part loves looking at these different areas of your life because this part only knows how to support and guide you to these experiences.

Now, with this list, I want you to number the priority of each. Perhaps getting a new job is number one, or perhaps leaving a negative relationship, or it could be losing weight successfully. The great thing about prioritising means that you are not trying to achieve everything at the one time. The Inner Critic loves you trying to do too much, so check in with yourself while going through your list: see it and yourself through the eyes of your Slim Confident part and see if what you have requested for yourself is manageable.

Now, as an exercise, I want you to look at the top two choices. How is it possible for these two areas of your life to come to fruition? Write down what needs to be done for just these two goals to be achieved. Remember: keep the Inner Critic out of your thoughts by continuing to release it on your out breath.

Visualising using all of your senses

With these two desires in your mind, I want you to find somewhere safe where you can sit or lie down and close your eyes. I want you to imagine what it feels like to have these two desires as part of your daily life. Daydream away with your senses and create as much colour and intensity as you need. Create what you are wearing, where you are and the people who are with you or, perhaps you are by yourself. Use all of your emotions of self love, excitement, desire and passion. Feel the warmth of the energy of seeing yourself in these situations. I want you to do this every day for the next month. It is your homework, so to speak. The more you do this, the easier it will become. I want you, when there is moment of self doubt, to recall these two goals and create them silently in your mind as many times as you possibly can, whether you are waiting in line at the supermarket or perhaps on a plane. Wherever and whenever, keep these two desires close to your heart and consistently experience them in your mind and heart.

Imagination and Reality

As the unconscious mind doesn't know the difference between imagination and reality you will, by doing this exercise every day, automatically be sending into your unconscious mind a real experience and it will take it on board as having already happened. The mind will then be driven by this desire because it thinks it is a normal way of thinking and it will work towards these goals automatically.

I use this technique with my clients all the time. Taking someone through this technique helps them gain confidence and a belief in self, whether it is weight loss or a fear of flying. The mind will take the information on board and will utilise it as part of the routine of where you are going in life. The mind is such a powerful tool, so never underestimate what you can accomplish through the power of your own mind. Thought does create reality and the more you imagine your future in this way the stronger the reality will be.

Whenever you experience any slight self doubt, bring these positive feelings on board. Remember to create what you are wearing, who is around you, what you are saying or doing. Please don't be squashed by negativity which creeps in: just keep repeating the image over again. Use every quiet time when it is available, whether waiting for the printer to finish or the washing machine, utilise every part of your day and night to build on these two wonderful goals.

The CD is a great way of doing this too. While listening to the CD you can just drift away or sometimes bring in these thoughts and memorise them so they are repeated over and over again while you are drifting away. Thought creates reality. This is your mind: no-one else but you can store these feelings for you. Visualise, feel, smell, taste and hear all of the images. Use energy in all of these creative thoughts. Remember: you have the right to be happy and this is the beginning of your imagination becoming reality.

This book is a reality now where once it was only a dream, and I remember being told by someone I trusted that I was a lousy writer - fortunately for me I didn't take what they said on board; however, I could have if my Confident Logical self hadn't known better. Thank goodness I had the belief and support of my literary agent and my family who have always said I had a story to tell. I dreamt of this moment, I saw my book, I saw the people in the workshops and it has become a reality.

You deserve to believe in yourself. You deserve to achieve what you want.

Your mind does, too, but you have to provide the information before it knows how to do it. Trust in this process and trust yourself. Remember, the past is the past. You are moving on from your past, through your present and into the future by the power of your own mind. This is your gift from you to you. Enjoy it!

Chapter 8

Protecting Yourself and Your Inner Dialogue

Your Conscious World

In order for you to continue feeling good about yourself and knowing that it is safe for you to have a healthy relationship with food, you will need to check in with your Inner Dialogue regularly. The CD, of course, is a great tool to enhance your positive Inner Dialogue but it is important also to respect your conscious world too.

Diarise your Inner Dialogue and the amazing array of emotions you are experiencing on a daily basis. Check in with yourself and ask yourself if you are feeling happy, sad, bored, tired or negative. Question why are you feeling this way? Perhaps someone has said something negative or perhaps you are feeling anxious about work. Are you feeling a desire to eat even though you know you are not hungry? Write down what is going on. It will help you in your understanding of how much your emotions and environment trigger certain binges.

A workshop participant once told me, "I didn't realise there was so much going on in my head. I feel for the first time in my life that I am the master of my own ship." The fact is, Inner Dialogue has always been there in our minds and always will be. The trick is how you manage 'it' rather than 'it' managing you. Being aware of your Inner Dialogue consciously allows you to make healthy decisions, rather than retreating back into old ways.

Step Outside Yourself

A great tool is to step outside yourself and think of yourself as being the judge of the jury. Through doing this, you will be able to assess the different opinions of your Inner Dialogue, then you will be able to make better-informed decisions of what you want and how you will accomplish this. Check in with all of the different options and notice which ones stir your feelings of vulnerability and which ones empower you. Most of the time, these stirrings are the left over residue of old fears and anxieties which have outlived their purpose.

Make an analysis of what you feel and be truthful within yourself about what is going on, rather than listening to the old Radio Crazy. Once again, write it down so you can see what is logical and what is not.

Apply yourself to think: if this situation was about someone else, what advice would you give them? This always brings an interesting response and will clear your decision-making process.

Start protecting yourself rather than everybody else, and utilise this time by seeing yourself through your Slim Confident part. How does your Slim Confident part react? What is the outcome you yourself want to achieve rather than your Pleaser, Perfectionist or any of the other parts? This is an exciting process, for there is always a positive outcome.

Other People's Approval

Other people can trigger anxiety when it comes to losing weight. As I have already mentioned, the Inner Critic will roll its eyes and issue the internal statement, "Here she/he goes again, another diet." Remember, you will always have to deal with the external comments of other people: that is a fact of life. However, you can change your own internal derogative comments.

Please remember that no-one can alleviate your anxiety about losing weight accept you. People may encourage or dismiss you and both can trigger an Inner Critic attack. The best solution is not to tell anybody. It truly isn't anybody else's business but yours. Whether they know or not that you want to lose weight or change your relationship with food, it is not going to make any difference. This is about you believing in you, and the power of knowing that you can rely on yourself emotionally means you don't need anybody else's approval.

There are many clients who say, "If I change how I eat people will notice, and I know immediately they will think I am on another diet and I get paranoid and scared, so I end up eating like I normally would."

My answer to that issue is to pretend you're not feeling well, or say something along the lines of: 'I don't think that agrees with me at the moment.' Most people will accept this statement and if they don't, then change the subject. Say things that appease yourself, so you feel safe to continue what you want to do rather than listening to your Inner Critic. This is a little white lie which will help support you with external comments.

External and Internal Critic Attacks

Jenny came to see me about her binge eating. She had read about my work through a magazine article and was desperate to lose weight. Jenny was doing really well during the weekdays, but weekends were proving a little more difficult for her. Jenny came from a background where Sunday lunches were still part of the family tradition. These family meals occurred two Sundays a month. It appeared that they were causing Jenny a lot of anxiety. We looked at the month that had just gone by and noticed that these binges directly correlated to these family moments.

I asked Jenny how she felt about these lunches and she replied, "I am the only single child left and the middle child. Both my brothers have been married for quite some time. It's not that they make me feel awful about being single, it's more the fact that they feel sorry for me and in fact I feel sorry for myself too. My mum goes on about my weight all the time. I always dread the 'how was your week?' question because it makes me feel so upset. I clench my teeth and smile but all I want to do is hide. I truly want to lose weight but every time I do, my mum comments, and then I feel like everybody is looking at me and I feel so awful I eat everything in sight, then I think: what's the point?"

I don't know how many times I have heard something similar to Jenny's story.

Other People's comments

Why is it that people feel the need to make comments on your weight every time they see you? This is one thing that really gets on my nerves. For me, it is a personal intrusion for someone to comment about your weight. I know the secret dieter within us always likes to know how someone has lost weight, but sometimes this can cause great emotional stirring and unnecessary stress. I used to dread losing weight because it was guaranteed someone would pipe up with: "Hey, Georgia – gosh, you've lost weight!" And I felt as if the whole room stopped and stared and I was on display like a piece of cattle to be sold at market.

When people do comment about your weight, immediately the Inner Critic says, "See? They thought you were fat all this time as they watched you gain weight and lose weight." Then there is the comment: "Hey, Georgia - you look well." What do they mean by that comment? My Inner Critic and many of my clients' Inner Critics interpret that comment as: 'they mean you have put on weight.' People don't seem to be able to stop making inane comments. It still baffles me why so many people think your body needs to be measured against the last time they saw you.

One of my friends once asked my professional advice regarding her cousin, who had put on a lot of weight. My friend asked whether I thought she should tell her, as the family had discussed how shocked they were with her sudden weight gain. I was extremely blunt to say the least and this is what I told her: "I appreciate that you are concerned but I don't think you need to tell her she has put on weight. Don't you think she knows she has put on all this weight?

Don't you think she goes to bed every night filled with anger and self loathing? Who do you think you are, suggesting that you need to tell her? Every time she dresses herself in the morning I guarantee she knows. Every time she has to buy the next size up pair of jeans she knows. If she wants to talk about it to you she will, and if she doesn't, that's her business. Just let her do it in her own time and if she doesn't want to lose weight, that is up to her."

I used to dread going home to Australia on my yearly visit because my Inner Critic would be waiting in the wings as the plane circled and landed at Melbourne airport. My Inner Dialogue ran through every conceivable comment just in case it happened, and the comments did happen from time to time. It's that not people want to be cruel: the sad fact is, people who don't have weight issues don't understand the complications and think they are being helpful, which they are not!

Once people comment about your weight loss or gain you can feel extremely exposed and vulnerable: this is normal and, of course, natural; however, their comments do not matter - it's your own inner comments that do. So don't listen to the never-ending Inner Critic chatter for its list just goes on and on. "Everybody else is watching you and your weight. Everybody knows you eat too much. People are more aware of you than you think."

Listening to this in itself triggers overeating because it stirs up anxiety and a sense of failure. I repeat: people, unfortunately, always seem to think they have the right to comment on your weight: this is sad but true and it is important when this occurs to protect yourself physically and emotionally, and the following advice will explain how you can accomplish this protection.

The Aura of Energy

Our body has an energy field surrounding us and this amazing field can assist us physically and intuitively. This energy field is referred to by some people as an aura. It is invisible to the eye but scientists now agree the aura field can be photographed through a certain type of camera.

If you were with me right now and you closed your eyes and I placed my hand approximately 10 centimetres away from your eyes, you probably wouldn't feel my hand. However, as I moved my hand closer at a certain point you would be able to feel the warm energy of my hand, and if you opened your eyes when you felt this energy my hand would be just a few centimetres away from your face. The reason you would feel this warm energy is because at that moment you would feel the sensation of the energy field, because your energy would have met with mine.

I demonstrate to clients the reality of this invisible field and so they can work with it to create a shield of protection in day to day life.

Why you need to shield yourself and The Shielding Tool

Wouldn't it be fabulous if you could lose weight safely without any of these insensitive comments infecting you? Well, you can! I am going to show you how to build a shield later on in this chapter.

Other people will always comment on your weight; however, until you feel strong enough to be more assertive there is a wonderful tool I give my clients to use when they need help to stay on track: I call it The Shielding Tool.

The fact is, you will need more shielding than ever as you lose weight because you will become more sensitive to people's comments. You need to be aware of this so you can continue to lose weight and reach the weight you desire. During this time you will need all the self protection you can get to enable you to get on with losing weight.

Negative People

There will always be someone waiting in the wings to bring you down when you achieve something good for yourself. Needless to say, it is a reflection of their own lack of self worth and unfortunately the world contains many negative people. The Shielding Tool will protect and prevent you from becoming infected by negative energy so you will be able to deal with unexpected or assumed external critic comments and continue to lose weight.

Certain people or situations you find yourself in will trigger a lack of confidence within you. Negative people have a nasty but clever habit of spotting someone's vulnerabilities and then playing on them, just like the Child Catcher in Chitty Chitty Bang Bang. These negative people can sense when a person has a particularly strong Pleaser. So be careful: use The Shielding Tool so you don't pick up their negative energy field. A negative person can transmit a negative energy field so make sure your shield is with you: protect yourself so you can be in the environment but not take their negative energy home with you. Sensing this negative energy in another means you are an intuitive person, so let's use this intuition to work with you.

During the last track on the CD I talk about the invisible energy field that surrounds you. Every person has this energy field and there will have been occasions when you have intuitively used yours. Think for a moment of a time when you found yourself in a situation where you have known the mood of a particular person even though they never uttered a word. In this situation, you picked up on their energetic field through your inbuilt sensing device and used your intuition.

The Shield of Weight

Some people create a shield of excess weight to protect themselves. As discussed in earlier chapters, the fear of sexual intimacy or avoiding getting on with life can be physically manifested in weight.

As you start to feel safer, you will notice that you don't need the protective layer of weight around your body. Start to transfer each pound you lose into your invisible shield, so you continue to feel safe but lighter and brighter physically and emotionally at the same time.

Take a deep look at what your true resistances are to losing the weight. Go back to your judge and jury and ask yourself the question: Why do I need to keep this weight on?

How to create your own special shield

Imagine a shield that envelops your physical body from head to toe and back to front. My shield will probably be different to yours and every else's, because we all have our own unique shield. Create your own shield through imagining what this protective layer feels and looks like. It may be a big golden light keeping you warm and safe in certain circumstances, or maybe it is plastic or glass armour, or a piece of satin or silk that wraps itself around you, keeping you safe. Imagine and create what suits you – experiment! There are no rules so relax and enjoy the process of creating your shield.

I take my shield everywhere with me. Whenever I feel a little bit scared, I wrap my shield around me so I feel safe in certain situations. It may be when I walk into a room and sense negativity, or it could be when I know in advance that I will need protection for the situation I will find myself in. For these advance situations, I always rehearse in the theatre of my mind the anticipated scene. Remember: your thoughts create reality. If there are times when you need extra protection, rehearse the scene in your mind before you go to sleep at night. Think about the outcome you want in this situation and how you will react. How do you want to feel before, during and after the event? Create and rehearse what you want to say in a calm, confident voice. See yourself and the positive outcome.

In the example of Jenny, her shield went with her to each family lunch and when her mother commented about her weight, she would politely reply, "Mum, does it really matter what weight I am? I am doing my best, please just let me get on with it." Jenny's courageous replies resulted in her mother backing down and Jenny achieved what she wanted: weight loss and respect. Remember, people only get away with hurtful behaviour and comments because we give them the power by allowing them to.

Energy

It takes a lot of energy to continue to lose weight, not to mention maintaining confidence and self belief. You must preserve your energy of confidence by keeping the shield in place when you find yourself in difficult situations, whether they be birthday parties, the pub or socialising at work functions. Eat what you want to eat and get on with it. If anybody comments, "Are you trying to lose weight?" say, "No": say anything and place your shield around you to keep you safe and protected.

If it is your partner, a family member or child who you feel gives you a hard time, reply: "I just feel like eating this." Remember, you are not on a diet - that is your old mentality.

Fiona's partner had issues with her weight loss. He and his Inner Critic didn't like Fiona losing weight because he was worried about her leaving. This relationship dynamic is more common than you may think. It was obvious after a month of hypnosis that Fiona had lost weight and of course her husband noticed, and he started bringing home chocolates and cakes for her to eat. Fiona had been through her husband's behaviour before whenever she had been on one of her previous diets. In order for Fiona to deal with this comfortably I said, "Instead of getting angry, talk to him about it and how you feel about the cake and chocolate. Remember to keep your shield around you."

Fiona's situation was a classic time for shielding, as it is often required with people you dearly love. They become frightened at the possibility of losing you when you become slim and confident, and their reaction is to protect themselves by doing things which undermine your keeping on track with your weight loss. I told Fiona to explain to him that her weight loss was important to her, that she needed to do this for herself and staying overweight would only increase her unhappiness, that this was not fair to her and his behaviour would only serve to destroy their relationship, not enhance it.

People ask other people to do things to hide their own insecurities. Don't sabotage your happiness for the sake of other people - after all, they are doing what they want, so why should you give in and stay the way you are in order to keep someone else happy? This is not the rule of fairness: everybody has the right to feel good about themselves.

While losing weight you need all the support and encouragement that you can receive from people who truly support you: these are the people with whom you don't need to keep your shield.

I can't stress enough how much The Shielding Tool is going to help you keep on track. Keep your shield around you during the situations when you need it, such as going for that important job interview or joining a new club. Remember: keep positive and protected when you need to.

Positive people and The Shielding Tool

The best thing about The Shielding Tool is that you become aware of when it is safe to let go of the shield and when it is not. You become more intuitive at assessing situations and the people who support you and those who don't.

Positive people pick up any signs of vulnerability and turn them into positives. So keep those positive people around you as an extra shield. As you do this, you will start to truly notice those who will help and guide you through good times and not-so-good times.

Being around positive people will enhance your success in building your self esteem and confidence, so please make time to enjoy the company of positive people. Remember, we are not as alone as we feel when we struggle with our weight.

You now have all of the tools you will need to keep yourself protected during all the moments while you are losing weight.

Track 3

You are now ready to listen to the final track on the CD. You can listen to all the tracks as much as you like. As you know, it doesn't matter whether you feel you have fallen asleep or not, it's all still being absorbed.

If you are short of time listen to track 1 on Monday, Tuesday track 2, Wednesday track 3 and then repeat. If your Inner Critic is particularly strong, listen to track 1, or if you are about to make a decision, track 3. However, they are all relevant to everyday life.

I hope you enjoy reading this book as much as I have enjoyed writing it. The words, emotions and knowledge expressed within these pages come with love, support and care.

Remember, your Slim Confident part is always with you through the thick and thin of life. Keep practising; it will get easier, more comfortable and natural and it will become automatic just like breathing. So take a big breath, begin and enjoy the process!

Take care.

Love,

Georgia

Bibliography, Further Reading and Resources

Georgia Foster can be contacted via her website:
www.georgiafoster.com

If you would like to attend a workshop in your area, please contact Georgia via her website. If you have 12 or more people, Georgia or one of her trainers would be delighted to come to you. Depending on location, travel expenses may be included over and above the cost of programme.

Complementary Health Clinics that Georgia works in are:
The Wren Clinic, Idol Lane, London EC3R 5DD
020 7283 8908 **www.wrenclinic.co.uk**

The Life Centre, 15 Edge Street, Notting Hill, London. W8 7PN
020 7221 4602 **www.thelifecentre.com**

Voice Dialogue books:
Stone, Hal and Sidra. Embracing Our Selves, Nataraj Publishing, 1989
Stone, Hal and Sidra. Embracing the Inner Critic, HarperSanFrancisco, 1993

For nutritional support and advice, please contact Gillian Hamer via The Wren Clinic at the above address.

"Gillian Hamer is a treasure. I can unreservedly recommend her both personally and professionally. She has helped me over illnesses of all kinds from debilitating flu to Post Traumatic Stress via candida and food sensitivities. As a journalist, I have also been very grateful for her expert advice, both for articles I have written for national newspapers and magazines, and also books...... Don't hesitate to consult her: you really won't regret it!"
Sarah Stacey
Health Editor, Mail On Sunday YOU magazine

For spiritual guidance, Hazel Oatey is an Energy/Crystal Practitioner. Hazel is available for private sessions and workshops around the UK. Contact her on; 07957 162 103 or by email; hazeloatey@yahoo.com

"I attended one of Hazel's workshops after my marriage broke up. I was searching for answers about my life. I feel so much more grounded and at peace now. I am more trusting about the flow of my life and have found a deeper level of understanding about myself."
Andrea, 35

Thanks to Amanda Seyderhelm, my writing coach and agent. The angels are with us. Amanda can be contacted on www.readytowrite.com

Carolyne Roberts, proof reader on demand, thanks for all your help. Carolyne can be contacted at NextDirection@aol.com.

Steve, you are the best book cover designer and typesetter. It's great working with such an optimistic person, thanks. Steve can be contacted at Steve@fever-design.co.uk.